PHARMACOLOGY - RESEARCH, SAFETY TESTING AND REGULATION

IMATINIB

CHEMICAL STRUCTURE, PHARMACOLOGY AND ADVERSE EFFECTS

PHARMACOLOGY - RESEARCH, SAFETY TESTING AND REGULATION

Additional books in this series can be found on Nova's website under the Series tab.

Additional e-books in this series can be found on Nova's website under the e-book tab.

CANCER ETIOLOGY, DIAGNOSIS AND TREATMENTS

Additional books in this series can be found on Nova's website under the Series tab.

Additional e-books in this series can be found on Nova's website under the e-book tab.

PHARMACOLOGY - RESEARCH, SAFETY TESTING AND REGULATION

IMATINIB

CHEMICAL STRUCTURE, PHARMACOLOGY AND ADVERSE EFFECTS

MOJTABA AKHTARI
AND
IHAB ELHEMAIDI
EDITORS

NOVA BIOMEDICAL

New York

For permission to use material from this book please contact us:
Telephone 631-231-7269; Fax 631-231-8175
Web Site: http://www.novapublishers.com

Library of Congress Cataloging-in-Publication Data

Library of Congress Control Number: 2013941196

ISBN: 978-1-62808-297-5

Published by Nova Science Publishers, Inc. † New York

Contents

Preface

Chronic myeloid leukemia (CML) has had a long lasting impact on modern medicine and the new era of targeted therapy. The causal link between cancer and genetic mutations was defined first in CML after the discovery of the Philadelphia chromosome in 1960 by Peter Nowell and David Hungerford. CML has always been at the forefront of a rapidly evolving field of hemato-oncology. More than 40 years on again CML stole the show by being the first cancer to have an FDA approved targeted novel molecular treatment in 2001 in the form of Imatinib which was developed by Nicholas Lydon, Brian Druker and Charles Sawyers. Imatinib has brought a revolution in the management of CML, a disease which had very limited therapeutic options including allogeneic hematopoietic stem cell transplantation and interferon-alpha 10 years ago. Imatinib is very active in CML, and it is associated with certain toxicities, which can be managed reasonably. The clinical success of imatinib in CML and gastrointestinal tumours (GIST) has brought up a new paradigm in cancer therapy that has very broad potentials. Imatinib is active against a number of related tyrosine kinases, namely ABL, BCR-ABL, KIT, PFGFR, and TEL. Now as more than a decade has passed since the approval of Imatinb and after the change of CML from a rapidly fatal disease to a more chronic and manageable disease we wanted to have a look back at what we know about the drug and its effect on various body systems. Its efficacy, side effect and how to manage its use in non-hematological malignancies is discussed in a detail. Gathering all this information in one book will be of immense benefit for healthcare workers including physicians, pharmacists and nurses and this in turn will help them improve the care of their patients. It will also be of benefit for pharmacists as a source of clinical and pharmacological knowledge. For researchers undertaking research in the field of hemato-oncology or pharmacology this will be a useful starting point for reviewing the literature. Imatinib is still being studied in patients in the clinic and laboratory models, and researchers are assessing the use of imatinib in other cancers. The editors have tried to allow information in book chapters to show different aspects and various view points on related issues. The editors have tried to get all the permissions before publication, and great attention has been spent in the preparation of this book. Having said that, however, mistakes cannot always be avoided. The editors and the publisher cannot accept responsibility for any errors that inadvertently happened. The opinions and views expressed in this volume are those of the participating authors and do not reflect the views of the editors, the publisher, or the manufacturer pharmaceutical product named herein. The current package insert should be consulted before any pharmaceutical product is used. We hope that our readers will find this book a useful and beneficial resourse in this complex and rapidly changing field in the new era of targeted therapy and renewed hope for cancer patients.

Mojtaba Akhtari

Ihab El-Hemaidi

Contributors

Pranab Sharma Acharya
Staten Island University Hospital, Staten Island,
New York, USA

Satoshi Akagi
Department of Cardiovascular Medicine,
Okayama University Graduate School of Medicine,
Dentistry and Pharmaceutical Sciences, Okayama, Japan

Mojtaba Akhtari
Division of Hematology and Oncology,
Department of Internal Medicine,
987680 Nebraska Medical Center,
University of Nebraska Medical Center, Omaha, NE,
68198-7680, USA, Mojtaba.akhtari@unmc.edu

Nicholas A Barber
Division of Hematology and Oncology,
Department of Internal Medicine,
University of Nebraska Medical Center,
987680 Nebraska Medical Center,
Omaha, NE, 68198-7680 USA

Vijaya Raj Bhatt
University of Nebraska Medical Center,
987680 Nebraska Medical Center, Omaha, NE,
68198-7680, USA

Jaurès Blanc
Innovation and Development Unit,
Service of Biomedicine,
Centre Hospitalier Universitaire Vaudois and University of Lausanne,
Lausanne, Switzerland

Thierry Buclin
Division of Clinical Pharmacology,
Service of Biomedicine,
Centre Hospitalier Universitaire Vaudois and University of Lausanne,
Lausanne, Switzerland

Chantal Csajka
Division of Clinical Pharmacology,
Service of Biomedicine,
Centre Hospitalier Universitaire Vaudois and University of Lausanne,
Lausanne, Switzerland; School of Pharmaceutical Sciences,
University of Geneva and University of Lausanne,
Geneva, Switzerland

Laurent A. Decosterd
Innovation and Development Unit,
Service of Biomedicine,
Centre Hospitalier Universitaire Vaudois and University of Lausanne,
Lausanne, Switzerland

Meekoo Dhar
Staten Island University Hospital, Staten Island,
New York, USA

Michel A. Duchosal
Service and Central Laboratory of Hematology,
Centre Hospitalier Universitaire Vaudois and University of Lausanne,
Lausanne, Switzerland

Ihab El-Hemaidi
Consultant Adult Hematology/BMT,
Princess Noorah Oncology Center,
Abdulaziz Medical City-Western Region,
National Guard Health Affairs, PO Box 9515,
eddah 21423, Kingdom of Saudi Arabia

Paolo Fava
Department of Biomedical Sciences and Human Oncology,
Section of Dermatology, University of Turin, v. Cherasco 23,
101026 Torino, Italia, tel. 011/6335816 - fax 011/6335034

Verena Gotta
Division of Clinical Pharmacology,
Service of Biomedicine, Centre Hospitalier Universitaire Vaudois and
University of Lausanne, Lausanne, Switzerland

Jun Guo
Department of Melanoma and Renal cancer,
Peking University Cancer Hospital and Institute,
Peking, China

Amina Haouala
Innovation and Development Unit,
Service of Biomedicine, Centre Hospitalier Universitaire Vaudois
and University of Lausanne, Lausanne, Switzerland

Hiroshi Ito
Department of Cardiovascular Medicine,
Okayama University Graduate School of Medicine,
Dentistry and Pharmaceutical Sciences, Okayama, Japan

Shiksha Kedia
Staten Island University Hospital,
Staten Island, New York, USA

Kusano Kengo
Department of Cardiovascular Medicine,
Okayama University Graduate School of Medicine,
Dentistry and Pharmaceutical Sciences, Okayama, Japan

Serge Leyvraz
Multidisciplinary Oncology Center, Centre Hospitalier Universitaire Vaudois
and University of Lausanne, Lausanne, Switzerland

Aurelio Lorico
Cancer Research Program, Roseman University of Health Sciences,
Las Vegas, NV, USA

Hiromi Matsubara
Division of Cardiology,
National Hospital Organization Okayama Medical Center,
Okayama, Japan

Kazufumi Nakamura
Department of Cardiovascular Medicine,
Okayama University Graduate School of Medicine,
Dentistry and Pharmaceutical Sciences, Okayama, Japan

Aiko Ogawa
Division of Cardiology, National Hospital Organization Okayama Medical Center,
Okayama, Japan

Manisha Pant
Jiri Hospital, Dolakha, Nepal

Germana Rappa
Cancer Research Program, Roseman University of Health Sciences,
Las Vegas, NV, USA

Paolo Savoia
Department of Biomedical Sciences and Human Oncology,
Section of Dermatology, University of Turin, v. Cherasco 23,
101026 Torino, Italia, tel. 011/6335816 - fax 011/6335034

Kate Vandyke
Myeloma Research Laboratory, Division of Haematology,
Centre for Cancer Biology, SA Pathology and School of Medicine,
University of Adelaide, Adelaide, Australia

Giuseppe Visani
Hematology and Hematopoietic Stem Cell Transplant Center,
AORMN Marche Nord, Pesaro, Italy

Nilakantan Viswanathan
Staten Island University Hospital, Staten Island,
New York, USA

Margaret von Mehren
Department of Medical Oncology, Fox Chase Cancer Center,
Philadelphia, Pennsylvania, USA

Nicolas Widmer
Division of Clinical Pharmacology,
Service of Biomedicine, Centre Hospitalier Universitaire Vaudois and
University of Lausanne,
Lausanne, Switzerland

Andrew C.W. Zannettino
Myeloma Research Laboratory, Division of Haematology,
Centre for Cancer Biology, SA Pathology and School of Medicine,
University of Adelaide,
Adelaide, Australia

In: Imatinib
Editors: Mojtaba Akhtari and Ihab Elhemaidi

ISBN: 978-1-62808-297-5

Chapter 1

The Chemical Structure, Pharmacology and Adverse Effects of Imatinib

Giuseppe Visani, Federica Loscocco, Teresa Ricciardi, Paola Picardi, Sara Barulli, Barbara Guiducci and Alessandro Isidori*

Hematology and Stem Cell Transplant Center,
AORMN Marche Nord, Pesaro, Italy

Abstract

Imatinib mesylate is a small molecule which acts by inhibiting enzymes with tyrosine kinase activity. Its molecular formula is C29H31N70 – CH4SO3 and its molecular weight is 493.603 g/mol. Imatinib mesylate is soluble in aqueous buffers ≤ pH 5.5 but is very slightly soluble to insoluble in neutral/alkaline aqueous buffers. Its mechanism of action is a competitive ATP inhibition at the catalytic binding site of abnormal tyrosine kinase created by the Philadelphia chromosome abnormality in chronic myeloid leukemia (CML) and in acute lymphoblastic leukemia (ALL). The BCR-ABL gene plays a central role in the pathogenesis of CML. In most cases, BCR-ABL is generated through reciprocal translocation between chromosomes 9 and 22 during formation of the Philadelphia chromosome (Ph). In normal cells, the ABL protein is located in the nucleus and its tyrosine kinase activity is strictly controlled, but in CML cells the BCR-ABL fusion protein is found in the cytoplasm and is constitutively active. Imatinib mesylate inhibits proliferation and induces apoptosis in bcr-abl positive cells. Nevertheless, Imatinib mesylate is also an inhibitor of the receptor tyrosine kinase for platelet-derived growth factor (PDGF), stem cell factor (SCF) and c-kit.

The pharmacological properties of Imatinib Mesylate show a mean absolute bioavailability of 98%. Following oral administration, the elimination half-life of imatinib and its major active metabolite, the N-demethil derivative (CGP74588), are 18 and 40 hours, respectively. CYP3A4 is the major enzyme responsible for metabolism of

* Address for correspondence: Hematology and Stem Cell Transplant Center, AORMN Marche Nord Via Lombroso, 1, 61100 Pesaro, Italy, Tel: +390721364039; E-mail: pesarohematology@yahoo.it.
Supported in part by AIL Pesaro Onlus.

imatinib. Therefore interactions are observed between imatinib and many agents inducing or inhibiting CYP3A or drugs metabolized by CYP3A4. The most common observed non haematologic adverse events reported are fluid retention (superficial edema or other fluid retention), nausea, diarrhea, muscle cramps, abdominal pain, musculoskeletal pain, rash. Most events are mild to moderate. Hematologic toxicity appears to be dependent on dose and disease type or disease stage. The incidence of severe cytopenia (grade III-IV according to NCI CTCAE V3.0) was 2 o 3 times higher in acute lymphoblastic leukemia (ALL) or in blast crisis and accelerated phase CML, with respect to chronic phase CML. Hematologic side effects include neutropenia, thrombocytopenia and anemia. The frequency of Grade 3 or 4 neutropenia and thrombocytopenia was between 2- and 3-fold higher in acute lymphoblastic leukemia (ALL) or in blast crisis and accelerated phase CML, with respect to chronic phase CML. The median duration of the neutropenic and thrombocytopenic episodes varied from 2 to 3 weeks, and from 2 to 4 weeks, respectively.

Introduction

Imatinib mesylate (formerly STI571) is a small molecule protein-tyrosine kinase inhibitor that strongly inhibits the activity of the BCR-ABL tirosine kinase (TK), as well as two receptor TKs: Kit, the receptor for stem cell factor (SCF) coded by the c-Kit proto-oncogene, and the platelet-derived growth factor receptors alpha and beta (PDGFR-α and PDGFR-β). TKIs are extensively metabolized by cytochrome P450 enzymes (CYP), whose activities are characterized by a large degree of interindividual variability. [1] Some TKIs are also substrates or inhibitors of the drug transporters P-glycoprotein (Pgp; coded by ABCB1) Breast Cancer Resistance Protein (BCRP; ABCG2) and the organic cation transporter 1 (hOCT1; SLC22A1). [2-5] A standard dosage can consequently produce extremely different circulating and cell concentration profiles from one patient to another, thus determining the selection of resistant cellular clones by low drug exposure or the occurrence of toxicity in case of over-exposure. [6] Identifying the best active and safe dosage for single patients to maximize therapeutic benefit has become a scientific and clinical challenge in the treatment armamentarium of both chronic myeloid leukemia (CML) and acute lymphoblastic leukemia (ALL). Imatinib is approved in numerous countries worldwide for the treatment of newly diagnosed Philadelphia chromosome-positive (Ph+) chronic- phase CML, Ph+ accelerated-phase or blast-crisis CML, in patients with Ph+ chronic-phase CML who have failed to respond to interferon-α therapy and in acute lymphoblastic leukemia patients. It is also indicated in paediatric patients with newly diagnosed Ph+ chronic-phase CML, in accelerated-phase or blast-crisis CML, or in chronic-phase CML after failure of interferon-α therapy or when the disease has recurred after haematopoietic stem cell transplantation (HSCT). [7, 8] Approved indications, however, may vary by country.

Chemical Structure and Pharmacology

Imatinib mesylate (C29H31N70.CH4SO3; MW 589.7) is a phenylaminopyrimidine derivate and is the 4-[(4-Methyl-1-piperazinyl)methyl]-N-[4-methyl-3-[[4-(3-pyridinyl)-2-pyrimid-inyl]amino]-phenyl]benzamidemethanesulfonate.

Imatinib is a protein-tyrosine kinase inhibitor, which potently inhibits the Abl tyrosine kinase at the *in vitro*, cellular, and *in vivo* level. The compound specifically inhibits proliferation of v-abl and bcr-abl expressing cells, suggesting it is not a wide-ranging antimitotic drug. [9] In colony formation assays, imatinib showed selective inhibition of Bcr-abl positive colonies. [10] In addition, imatinib is a potent inhibitor of Arg, the platelet-derived growth factor receptor (PDGF-R), c-Kit, the receptor for SCF, and c-Fms, the receptor for macrophage-stimulating factor (M-CSF). [10, 11] In contrast, it does not affect signal transduction mediated by other *stimuli* comprising epidermal growth factor, insulin and phorbol ester. *In vivo*, Imatinib shows anti-tumor properties as a single agent in animal models at well tolerated doses. [10, 11]

Toxicology

Repeat-dose oral toxicology studies were performed in rats (up to 26 weeks), dogs (up 13 weeks) and monkeys (up to 39 weeks). [9-13] The no toxic effects levels (NTELs) were 5 mg/kg and 15 mg/kg at 26 weeks in rats and at 13 weeks in monkeys, respectively. In the 13-week study in dogs, the NOAEL (no observed adverse effect level) was 3 mg/kg. [9-13] In a 39-week monkey study, no NOAEL (no observed adverse effect level) was established at the lowest dose of 15 mg/kg, approximately one-third the maximum human dose of 800 mg based on body surface. [9-13]

Mild to moderate hematological changes occurred in rats, dogs and monkeys at oral doses ≥ 20, 10 and 75 mg/kg, respectively. Atrophy of lymphoid organs and lymphoid depletion were observed at oral doses ≥ 200 mg/kg in rats and ≥ 30 mg/kg in dogs. Emesis occured at oral doses of ≥ 30 mg/kg in dogs and ≥ 75 mg/kg in monkeys. [9-13] In the dog, diarrhea was observed at oral doses ≥ 3 mg/kg/day and a reduction in spermatogenesis at doses ≥ 30 mg/kg. The liver was a target organ in rats and dogs. [9-13] Mild to moderate increases in transaminases and slight decreases in cholesterol, triglycerides, total protein and albumin levels were observed in both species. No histopathological changes were seen in rat liver. Severe liver toxicity was observed in dogs treated for 2 weeks, with elevated liver enzymes, hepatocellular necrosis, bile duct necrosis, and bile duct hyperplasia. Renal toxicity was observed in monkeys treated for 2 weeks, with focal mineralisation and dilation of the renal tubules and tubular nephrosis. [9-13] Increased blood urea nitrogen (BUN) and creatinine were observed in several of these animals. [9-13] In rats, hyperplasia of the transitional epithelium in the renal papilla and in the urinary bladder was observed at doses of 6 mg/kg in the 13-week study, without changes in serum or urinary parameters. An increased rate of opportunistic infections was observed with chronic imatinib treatment. [9-13] The pharmacological effects of imatinib on its different molecular targets can be an explanation of the effects of the compound on lymphoid tissue, bone marrow and testis. [9-13]

Imatinib is not a mutagen but a teratogenic effect was observed in rats at doses of ≥ 100 mg/kg. Imatinib was teratogenic in rats when administered during organogenesis at doses ≥ 100 mg/kg, [12, 13] approximately equal to the maximum clinical dose of 800 mg/day, based on body surface area. [12, 13] Teratogenic effects included exencephaly or encephalocele, absent/reduced frontal and absent parietal bones. These effects were not seen at doses ≤ 30 mg/kg.

Imatinib was not considered genotoxic when tested in an in vitro bacterial cell assay (Ames test), an in vitro mammalian cell assay (mouse lymphoma) and an in vivo rat micronucleus test. [12, 13] Positive genotoxic effects were obtained for imatinib in an in vitro mammalian cell assay (Chinese hamster ovary) for clastogenicity (chromosome aberration) in the presence of metabolic activation. [12, 13]

The fertility of male and female rats was not affected, though there was decreased spermatogenesis in dogs and rats. [14, 15] In fact, the tyrosine kinase receptor c-kit and its interaction with the ligand, stem cell factor (SCF), play an essential role in the developing testis. [14, 15] C-kit is important for the development of the Leydig cells and for the migration, proliferation and survival of spermatogonia. Platelet-derived growth factor (PDGF) and its tyrosine kinase receptor (PDGFR) are important for the development of Leydig cells and myoid cells. Imatinib inhibits both of these tyrosine kinase receptors. [16] Three-day treatment of immature male rats (SD) with imatinib (150 mg/kg) on postnatal days 5-7 delayed the formation of germ-line stem cell pool, reduced proliferation of type A spermatogonia and induced germ cell apoptosis. [14, 15] PDGFR-mediated proliferation of mesenchymal myoid precursors was also decreased and the length of the seminiferous cord was reduced [14, 15]. However, at the age of 11 weeks the exposed animals had normal epididymal sperm counts, whereas plasma levels of luteinizing hormone and follicle stimulating hormone were significantly increased. [14, 15] Increased post-implantation loss was observed in the fertility study with treatment of both males and females, and in the embryotoxicity study with the treatment of females. Consequently, imatinib is considered embryoletal at high doses. [14, 15]

Pharmacokinetics and Drug Metabolism

Imatinib is well absorbed and rapidly cleared in all investigated species. [6, 12, 13, 17] Tissue distribution of imatinib and its metabolites was extensive and displayed reversible affinity to melanin-containing tissue, e.g. skin, ocular membranes and hair. Protein binding was moderate and differed between laboratory species and humans. [6, 12, 13, 17] Following oral administration in healthy volunteers, the t½ was approximately 18 h, suggesting that once-daily dosing is appropriate. [6, 12, 13, 17] The increase in mean AUC with increasing dose was linear and dose proportional in the range of 25–1000 mg imatinib after oral administration. [6, 12, 13, 17] There was no change in the kinetics of imatinib on repeated dosing, and accumulation was 1.5–2.5-fold at steady state when dosed once daily. [6, 12, 13, 17]

Imatinib is a substrate for CYP3A4 and is a competitive inhibitor of CYP3A4, whereas CYP1A2, CYP2D6, CYP2C19 CYP2C9 and CYP3A5 are reported to play a minor role in its metabolism. [1, 6, 12, 13] This TKI has also been shown to be a substrate for hOCT1, Pgp and BCRP. [3, 4, 18] However, another report suggests that imatinib is an inhibitor and not a substrate of BCRP, thus leaving ambiguity about the function of this pathway. [19]

In men, mean absolute imatinib bioavailability was 98%. [12, 13, 20] In the dose range between 25 and 1000 milligrams (oral administration), the increase in area under the curve (AUC) was linear and dose proportional.

Accumulation was about 1.5 to 3 fold (at steady state) when dosed once daily, and no change was observed in kinetics when administered in repeated dosing. [12, 13, 20]

Only 13% of imatinib was excreted in the urine. The PK profile was unaffected by age and gender. [20] The major metabolite identified in plasma (CGP74588) is pharmacologically active with similar potency to imatinib. [6, 12, 13] The metabolites of imatinib are eliminated predominantly through biliary excretion. One metabolite, an N-demethylated piperizine derivative (CGP 74588) shows pharmacologic activity comparable to the parent drug, but the systemic exposure represents ~ 15% of that for imatinib. [6, 12, 13] The fecal-to-urinary excretion ratio is ~ 5:1. Moreover, imatinib can competitively inhibit the metabolism of drugs that are CYP2C9, CYP2C19, CYP2D6, and CYP3A4 substrates. Imatinib is ~ 95% bound to human plasma proteins, mainly albumin and α1-acid glycoprotein. [6, 12, 13, 20-22]

Interactions should therefore be considered when administering inhibitors of the CYP3A family in combination with imatinib. [1, 23] A single dose of ketoconazole increased mean C_{max} and AUC of imatinib by 26% and 40%, respectively, confirming that imatinib is a CYP3A4 substrate. [24] Interactions are likely to occur with other inhibitors of CYP3A4, such as levothyroxine, voriconazole, or amiodarone, leading to an increase in plasma concentrations of imatinib. Nonetheless, Imatinib increased the C_{max} and AUC of simvastatin by 2- and 3.5-fold, respectively, indicating inhibition of CYP3A4. [1, 23] Co-administration with rifampin, an inducer of CYP3A4, reduced plasma imatinib AUC by approximately 70%. Acute dosing of ritonavir, as reviewed by Foisy did not change steady-state exposure to imatinib, but increased exposure to the major metabolite CGP74588 by > 40%. [25]

Simultaneous administration of Imatinib with inhibitors of both CYP3A4 and Pgp increase both plasma and intracellular imatinib concentrations. [24, 26] Dual inhibitors of CYP3A4 and Pgp such as ketoconazole, fluconazole, itraconazole, ciclosporin, erythromycin, clarithromycin and verapamil, raise intracellular concentrations of Imatinib by inhibition of both its metabolism and its efflux (through Pgp) and could as a result boost its cellular toxicity. [1, 6, 12, 13, 24, 26, 27]

Concurrent administration of CYP3A4 inducers such as rifampicin or some antiepileptics could determine a reduction of as much as 74% in imatinib exposure. [6, 12, 13] Furthermore, the imatinib pharmacokinetic profile was significantly modified by St John's wort, with reductions of 30% in the median AUC. [28, 29] Concomitant use of enzyme inducers, including St John's wort, may possibly necessitate an increase in imatinib dosages to preserve clinical efficacy. [28, 29]

Interactions between Imatinib and inhibitors of hOCT1 such as ranitidine, quinidine, or midazolam, could paradoxically raise the imatinib circulating concentrations but reduce the intracellular exposure of target cancer cells that express this carrier too. [6, 12, 13, 30]

Pertaining to all these mechanisms, it is important to keep in mind that plasma concentrations of imatinib seem to be correlated with imatinib efficacy and toxicity. A change in imatinib exposure caused by a drug interaction could therefore absolutely influence its therapeutic efficacy.

TKIs are also responsible for the inhibition of drug transporters and enzymes, leading to alterations in the exposure and consequently therapeutic effects of co-administered drugs. This is worth recalling for drug such as cyclosporin, a CYP3A4 and Pgp substrate, which is more adsorbed when co-administerd with Imatinib. [23, 27] Simultaneous administration of Imatinib may therefore increase the pharmacologic effects and possibly toxicity of ciclosporin.

Nonetheless, administration of imatinib together with metoprolol, a CYP2D6 substrate, resulted in an increase in metoprolol exposure by 23%. Finally, the clearance of simvastatin (a CYP3A4 substrate) was reduced by 70% when associated with imatinib. [12, 13, 23]

Interactions between Imatinib and calcium channel blockers substrates of CYP3A4 such as verapamil and diltiazem may cause an increase in the circulating levels of these drugs. Interactions with quinidine, amiodarone, and simvastatin, substrates for the same P450 isoenzyme, could as well be of clinical significance. [23] In patients taking imatinib, these drugs should be avoided and substituted with safer alternatives (e.g. pravastatin or sotalol).

As a matter of fact, it has been reported that inhibits the O-glucuronidation of acetaminophen, leading to hepatotoxicity and liver failure. [12, 13] Therefore, the use of acetaminophen should be limited or avoided in patients receiving imatinib; a limit of 1300 mg acetaminophen per day has been suggested, without a clear evidence of safety for this dosage. Liver function tests might be used to monitor prolonged treatment. [31] Acenocoumarol and phenprocoumon, substrates of CYP2C9, show also increased concentrations. However, this interaction can be compensated by the monitoring of prothrombin time or international normalized ratio.

Data concerning interactions involving protein binding are poorly documented for imatinib.

Finally, patients with hypothyroid conditions who receive imatinib need increased levothyroxine doses, probably due to an induction of non–deiodination clearance. [32] The part of levothyroxine that is deiodinated into triiodothyronine is primarily subject to conjugation with glucuronates and sulfates. Although the liver primarily mediates glucuronidation and sulfation, these conjugations occur in extrahepatic sites as well (e.g kidneys and intestine).

Therefore, induction of uridine diphosphate–glucuronyl transferases (UGTs) seems to be involved. For patient starting imatinib, a 2-fold increase in levothyroxine substitution therapy is recommended, together with close monitoring of thyroid function.

As in adult patients, imatinib is rapidly absorbed after oral administration in children. There was considerable inter-patient variability in the PK parameters. Imatinib exposure in children at 260 and 340 mg/m^2 was similar to doses of 400 mg and 600 mg in adult patients, respectively. [20]

Physical, Chemical and Pharmaceutical Properties

The molecular formula of Imatinib is $C_{29}H_{31}N_7O.CH_4SO_3$. Its relative molecular mass is 493.6 + 96.1 = 589.7. The molecule is not chiral. Imatinib is very or freely soluble in water and aqueous solutions at low pH levels.

The solution tends to become supersaturated. The solubility in an aqueous buffer solution drops to "insoluble" as the pH increases from pH 5.5 to 8.0. Imatinib is soluble in polar solvents such as methanol and ethanol but only slightly soluble or insoluble in low polar solvents. [12, 13]

Dissociation constant (pKa): Three pKa values were determined by potentiometric titration in a system dioxane/water at 25.0°C in 0.15 mol/L KCl. The pKa values are: 7.8, 3.8 and 3.3. [12, 13]

Cellular Profile of Imatinib

Imatinib was assayed in cellular system to evaluate its specificity and mechanism of action. Imatinib inhibited autophosphorylation of v-abl as well as p210bcr-abl, p185bcr-abl and TEL-abl fusion proteins with $IC5_0$ values between 0.1-0.35 μM. [9-11, 33] Inhibition of abl tyrosine kinase activity was also found in p210bcr-abl-positive myeloid and p185bcr-abl-positive lymphoblastic leukemia cell lines, as well as in leukemic cells obtained from patients with Ph+ CML and ALL. [9-11, 33]

Adverse Effects

Imatinib mesylate is associated with mild to moderate toxicity, mostly reversible by dose reduction or discontinuation of the drug. Most adverse effects occur within the first 2 years of starting therapy; however, late effects, many being unique, are now being recognized.

First of all, we will focus on data from the phase III IRIS study of patients with chronic-phase CML and from the most relevant phase II studies in patients with accelerated-phase or blast-crisis CML or those who had failed prior therapy with interferon-alpha as reported in the manufacturer's prescribing information and in the 60-months update from the IRIS study. [12, 13, 34, 35, 36] In these studies, adverse events were classified according to US National Cancer Institute Common Toxicity Criteria (CTC).

The vast majority of patients who received imatinib in these studies experienced adverse events, mostly of mild to moderate severity, at some time during the studies. Overall, the most common adverse events occurring in at least one third of patients with chronic-phase CML who received first line treatment in the IRIS study were: superficial oedema (58%), nausea (47%), muscle cramps (43%), muskoskeletal pain (39%), diarrhea (39%), cutaneous rash (37%), fatigue (37%) and headache (34%). [34] No statistical significance between patients receiving imatinib or cytarabine and alpha-interferon was reported. CTC grade 3 and 4 adverse events were less common in patients receiving imatinib with respect to patients receiving cytarabine and alpha-interferon. [34]

Long-term adverse event data from the phase III study showed a similar profile of adverse events reported earlier, but with a median follow-up of 60 months. The most common adverse events in patients with chronic-phase CML receiving Imatinib in the IRIS study were: oedema (60%), nausea (50%), muscle cramps (49%), muskoskeletal pain (47%), diarrhea (45%), cutaneous rash and other skin problems (40%), fatigue (39%) and headache (37%). Other common adverse events were abdominal pain (37%) and joint pain (31%). [35]

Grade 3 or 4 events were mainly hematological. Grade 3 or 4 neutropenia, thrombocytopenia or anemia occurred in imatinib recipients in all phase II and the phase III studies. The incidence of hematological grade 3 or 4 adverse effects was higher in patients with accelerated-phase or blast-crisis CML than in those with chronic-phase CML (first- or second-line treatment). [35] Patients receiving imatinib presented a significantly lower incidence of grade 3 plus 4 neutropenia (12+3%, $p<0.001$) and thrombocytopenia (8+0.2%, $p<0.001$) than patients receiving interferon plus cytarabine in the IRIS study. [35] The median duration of neutropenic episodes was 2-3 weeks and that of thrombocytopenic episodes was 2-4 weeks.

Hematological toxicity is managed by reducing the imatinib dosage or discontinuing treatment until resolution of the event (see manufacturer's prescribing information for dosage reduction recommendations). [12, 13, 35, 36]

About 5% of all patients with CML develop mild (grade 1/2) hepatotoxicity characterized by an abnormal bilirubin and transaminases within the first 2 years of receiving imatinib. [12, 13, 35, 36] Serious hepatotoxicity (grade 3/4) is, however, extremely rare. [12, 13, 35, 36] In all cases, the hepatic dysfunction appears to be fully reversible with dose interruption/dose reduction.

Cutaneous reactions are probably TKI-class related and are developed in different grades in several patients with CML on imatinib. [37] The exact incidence of rashes appears to be around 35%, mostly associated with pruritus.

A correlation between imatinib dosages and cutaneous reactions has not been clearly demonstrated; the vast majority of rashes develop during the initial 3 months of imatinib treatment. [37] Severe life-threatening exfoliative dermatitis and Stevens–Johnsons syndrome have also been reported rarely and have generally occurred within 10 days of starting therapy. [38] Approximately in 70-80% of the patients the rash and pruritus fall down significantly with treatment interruption alone; however, the addition of a short course of steroids is helpful. [37]

Kerkela et al. [39] reported their single centre experience on 10 patients who developed severe congestive heart failure while on imatinib and showed that imatinib-treated mice developed left ventricular contractile dysfunction. The authors demonstrated that with imatinib treatment, cardiomyocytes show in culture activation of the endoplasmic reticulum (ER) stress response, collapse of the mitochondrial membrane potential, release of cytochrome C into the cytosol, reduction in cellular ATP content and cell death. [39]

Retroviral gene transfer of an imatinib-resistant mutant of c-abl, alleviation of ER stress or inhibition of Jun amino-terminal kinases, which are activated as a consequence of ER stress, largely rescues cardiomyocytes from imatinib-induced death.

Thus, the authors postulated that cardiotoxicity is an unanticipated side effect of inhibition of c-abl by imatinib. However, many of these patients might have pre-existing conditions that predisposed them to CHF, and the authors admitted that the risk of CHF with Imatinib could not be precisely defined with this study. [39-43]

In vitro studies have suggested that imatinib may be toxic to cardiac myocytes. [12, 13] However, retrospective studies have not shown clinical heart failure; nevertheless, these studies did not look for subtle cardiac damage. Estabragh et al carried out a prospective cardiac assessment in 59 CML patients treated with imatinib for a median of 3.4 years, using echocardiography and MUGA scanning, with the latter repeated after a further year. [44] The Authors reported no evidence of myocardial deterioration, either at baseline or over 12 months of imatinib treatment. [44] Imatinib cardiotoxicity was not reported as an important clinical consideration for CML patients or their advisors. [40]

However, the US prescribing information reported on a case of one patient with blast-crisis CML who died with pleural effusion, congestive heart failure and renal failure, and the 60-months follow-up of the IRIS trial also reported 1 patient(<1%) with drug-related CHF. A follow-up examination of the Novartis database of imatinib clinical trials, including several different indications, spanning over 5600 years of patients exposure to imatinib found that the incidence of CHF in imatinib recipients was 0.2% cases per year with a possible or probable relationship to the drug. [12, 13]

The incidence of cardiac failure and left ventricular dysfunction in the IRIS study was estimated at 0.04% per year in the imatinib group versus 0.75% per year in interferon-alpha plus cytarabine recipients. [34-36] Other cardiac adverse effects include pericarditis, tachycardia, hypertension, and hypotension and collectively the incidence appears less than 1.0%. [34-36] It seems reasonable to state that, based on currently available evidence, cardiac toxicity does not appear to be a significant risk factor of long-term imatinib (IM) therapy. It will, however, appear prudent to remain vigilant. Clearly, patients with a pre-existing cardiac problem should be observed very closely and if signs of cardiac dysfunction develop, alternative treatment should be considered.

Several efforts have been made to study the effect of imatinib on bone and mineral metabolism. [45-52] The most relevant study was conducted by Berman et al. [45] A significant number of patients receiving imatinib for either GIST or CML developed hypophosphatemia with associated bone and mineral metabolic changes. The authors theorized that abnormalities in bone and mineral metabolism may be developed not only as a consequence of hypophosphatemia, but also as a direct result of inhibiting the PDGF-R. [45] Furthermore, it has also been advised using prospectively collected data that in the early stages of imatinib therapy may occur altered bone remodeling and secondary hyperparathyroidism. Imatinib could directly stimulate osteoblast bone building activity and limit osteoclast bone resorption activity, resulting in a flux of calcium from extracellular fluid into bone, a decreased serum calcium level, and a compensatory rise in the level of parathyroid hormone, thus leading to phosphaturia and hypophosphatemia. [46-52] More recently, an Italian group evaluated the effects of imatinib on osteoblastic differentiation of human bone marrow mesenchymal stem cells (hBM-MSCs). After 21 days of culture, hBM-MSCs treated with IM (1 microM) alone or osteogenic medium (OM) + IM showed changes in morphology with evidence of extracellular mineralization and increased mRNA expression of osteogenic markers, such as RUNX2, osteocalcin (OCN), and bone morphogenetic protein (BMP-2). [47] In summary, this paper showed that imatinib increases mRNA expression of osteogenic markers in hBM-MSCs and increases the OPG/RANKL ratio and the OCN levels both in supernatant of hBM-MSCs cultured with IM and in serum of patients treated with IM, thus indicating that IM potentially favors osteoblastogenesis. [47]

The long term effects of IM therapy on bone remodeling were also studied. Fitter et al. [48] evaluated the effect of long-term therapy on osteoblastic function in an attempt to evaluate the effects of imatinib on skeletal metabolism.

This was done by performing a pre- and (2–4 year) post-treatment analysis on patients' bone marrow. Half the patients (8 of 17) showed a substantive increase in total bone volume (TBV) (> 2-fold), after imatinib therapy, with the TBV in the post-treatment biopsy typically surpassing the normal upper limit for the patient's age group. Imatinib-treated patients exhibited reduced serum calcium and phosphate levels with hypophosphatemia evident in 53% (9 of 17) of patients. [48] The authors speculated that imatinib restrains bone resorption (by inhibiting c-Fms on osteoclasts) and stimulates bone formation (by inhibiting PDGF-R on osteoblasts), thus sequestrating both calcium and phosphate in bone. This can result in secondary hyperparathyroidism, which decreases renal phosphate absorption, leading to hypophosphatemia. [48]

At present, the clinical implications of the studies cited above are limited. Even if it appears that checking phosphorous and vitamin D levels over time may be logical, further studies are warranted, mainly to determine the long-term effects.

The Société Française des Cancers de l'enfant (SFCE) recently published the results of an open-label, multicentric phase IV trial evaluating the efficacy and safety of imatinib in children and adolescents with untreated CML, and confirmed a statistically significant decrease of height in half of the study patients (22/44). This negative impact of IM on skeletal growth also merits further study. [53]

The management of patients with chronic myeloid leukemia (CML) during pregnancy is a matter of continued debate. [54-56] The introduction of the TKIs in clinical practice has dramatically changed the prognosis of CML patients. Patients diagnosed in chronic phase can reasonably expect many years of excellent disease control and good quality of life. In view of this fact it has become a necessity to address issues relating to fertility and pregnancy. Physicians are not infrequently being asked for advice regarding the need for, and or the appropriateness of, stopping treatment in order to conceive.

The management of fertility begins at diagnosis. This means that immediate and future treatments should be considered at the very beginning of the treatment. Therefore, the maintenance of fertility should be taken in account since the diagnosis.

Imatinib is not genotoxic but might lead to a decrease in sperm counts. [12, 13] Nevertheless, Imatinib is teratogenic in rats when given during organogenesis at doses >100 mg/kg, approximately equivalent to 800 mg/day in men. [12, 13] Until now, approximately 60 pregnancies were reported in partners of men on Imatinib. [12, 13] No suggestions of any problems in conception, pregnancy, delivery or of any increase in congenital abnormalities were reported. [12, 13]

A small study from Houston in 2006 described outcomes of pregnancies in 19 patients undergoing treatment with IM. It is of interest that this study assessed 10 females and 8 males whose partners were pregnant. IM therapy was discontinued in all female patients immediately following the confirmation of pregnancy. [54] The majority of patients conceived without complication, and the authors concluded that conception among patients with CML receiving IM can ultimately lead to normal pregnancies, but given the low number of patients, an effect on miscarriages and birth abnormalities could not be ruled out. [54]

Regarding women, 204 patients were exposed to Imatinib, and 180 were reported in literature (76, 77). [55] Of 180 women exposed to imatinib during pregnancy, outcome data are available for 125 (69%).

Of those with known outcomes, 50% delivered normal infants and 28% underwent elective terminations, 3 following the identification of abnormalities. There were a total of 12 infants in whom abnormalities were identified, 3 of which had strikingly similar complex malformations that are clearly a cause for concern. [55] It appears that although most pregnancies exposed to imatinib are likely to have a successful outcome, there remains a risk that exposure may result in serious fetal malformations. [54] Although numbers are small there has been a disturbing cluster of rare congenital malformations such that imatinib cannot be safely recommended, particularly during the period of organogenesis. [12, 13] Last but not least, it has recently been reported a poor outcome after reintroduction of Imatinib in patients who interrupt therapy for pregnancy without having achieved an optimal response, introducing another variable in the management of women pregnant while receiving Imatinib. [56]

It is, therefore, prudent to advise female patients to avoid conception while on IM. Parenthetically, it should be noted that since IM is secreted in breast milk, breastfeeding is not recommended while on IM. [12, 13]

Current evidence does not suggest a congenital risk in male patients who are on imatinib at time of their partner conceiving, but it would appear reasonable to remain cautious. Oligospermia and reduced sperm motility have been observed in animals and humans treated with imatinib. [12, 13] A potential option might be to cryopreserve sperms prior to starting therapy with imatinib.

The above findings reveals a number of issues in evaluating the toxicities of a relative young drug. A number of findings that are present in the preclinical setting are not always apparent in the clinical setting, and vice versa. Outstandingly, after a decade of everyday use of imatinib in the clinical setting, the safety analysis suggests that the short [34, 35] and long-term [36, 57, 58] adverse effects of imatinib are quite acceptable.

References

[1] Van Erp, N. P., Gelderblom, H., Karlsson, M. O., et al. Influence of CYP3A4 inhibition on the steady-state pharmacokinetics of imatinib. *Clin. Cancer Res.* 2007;13(24):7394-7400.

[2] Ozvegy-Laczka, C., Hegedus, T., Varady, G., et al. High-affinity interaction of tyrosine kinase inhibitors with the ABCG2 multidrug transporter. *Mol. Pharmacol.* 2004;65(6): 1485-1495.

[3] Breedveld, P., Pluim, D., Cipriani, G., et al. The effect of Bcrp1 (Abcg2) on the in vivo pharmacokinetics and brain penetration of imatinib mesylate (Gleevec): implications for the use of breast cancer resistance protein and P-glycoprotein inhibitors to enable the brain penetration of imatinib in patients. *Cancer Res.* 2005;65(7):2577-2582.

[4] Brendel, C., Scharenberg, C., Dohse, M., et al. Imatinib mesylate and nilotinib (AMN107) exhibit high-affinity interaction with ABCG2 on primitive hematopoietic stem cells. *Leukemia* 2007;21(6):1267-1275.

[5] Melo, J. V. Imatinib and ABCG2: who controls whom? *Blood* 2006;108(4):1116-1117.

[6] Van Erp, N. P., Gelderblom, H., Guchelaar, H. J. Clinical pharmacokinetics of tyrosine kinase inhibitors. *Cancer Treat. Rev.* 2009;35(8):692-706.

[7] Novartis Pharmaceuticals Corporation. Prescribing information (US): Gleevec® (imatinib mesylate) tablets [online]. Available from URL: http://www.fda.gov/Drugs/default.htm [Accessed 2012 Jul 25]

[8] Novartis Europharm Limited. Prescribing information (EU): Glivec® (imatinib mesylate) tablets [online]. Available from URL: http://www.emea.europa.eu/ema/index.jsp?curl=pages/medicines/human/medicines/000406/human_med_000808.jsp [Accessed 2012 Jul 25]

[9] Druker, B. J., Tamura, S., Buchdunger, E., et al. Effects of a selective inhibitor of the Abl tyrosine kinase on the growth of Bcr-abl positive cells. *Nat. Med.* 1996 May; 2(5): 561-6.

[10] Druker, B. J., Lydon, N. B. Lessons learned from the development of an abl tyrosine kinase inhibitor for chronic myelogenous leukemia. *J. Clin. Invest.* 2000 Jan.;105(1):3-7.

[11] Druker, B. J. Perspectives on the development of a molecularly targeted agent. *Cancer Cell.* 2002;1(1):31-36.

[12] Glivec® (imatinib) summary of product characteristics. West Sussex, UK: Novartis Europharm Limited; 2010.
[13] Glivec® (imatinib) summary of product characteristics. West Sussex, UK: Novartis Europharm Limited; 2012.
[14] Nurmio, M., Toppari, J., Zaman, F., et al. Inhibition of tyrosine kinases PDGFR and c-kit by imatinib mesylate interferes with postnatal testicular development in the rat. *Int. J. Androl.* 2007; 30(4): 366-376.
[15] Nurmio, M., Kallio, J., Toppari, J., Jahnukainen, K. Adult reproductive functions after early postnatal inhibition by imatinib of the two receptor tyrosine kinases, c-kit and PDGFR, in the rat testis. *Reprod. Toxicol.* 2008; 25(4): 442-446.
[16] Buchdunger, E., Cioffi, C. L., Law, N., et al. The Abl protein-tyrosine kinase inhibitor, STI 571, inhibits in vitro signal transduction mediated by c-Kit and PDGF receptors. *J. Pharmacol. Exp. Ther.* 2000; 295: 129-145.
[17] Widmer, N., Decosterd, L. A., Leyvraz, S., et al. Relationship of imatinib-free plasma levels and target genotype with efficacy and tolerability. *Br. J. Cancer* 2008; 98(10): 1633-1640.
[18] White, D. L., Saunders, V. A., Dang, P., et al. OCT-1-mediated influx is a key determinant of the intracellular uptake of imatinib but not nilotinib (AMN107): reduced OCT-1 activity is the cause of low in vitro sensitivity to imatinib. *Blood* 2006; 108 (2): 697-704.
[19] Houghton, P. J., Germain, G. S., Harwood, F. C., et al. Imatinib mesylate is a potent inhibitor of the ABCG2 (BCRP) transporter and reverses resistance to topotecan and SN-38 in vitro. *Cancer Res.* 2004; 64(7):2333-2337.
[20] Petain, A., Kattygnarath, D., Azard, J., et al. Population pharmacokinetics and pharmacogenetics of imatinib in children and adults. *Clin. Cancer Res.* 2008;14(21): 7102-7109.
[21] Widmer, N., Decosterd, L. A., Csajka, C., et al. Population pharmacokinetics of imatinib and the role of alpha-acid glycoprotein. *Br. J. Clin. Pharmacol.* 2006;62(1):97-112.
[22] Azuma, M., Nishioka, Y., Aono, Y., et al. Role of alpha1-acid glycoprotein in therapeutic antifibrotic effects of imatinib with macrolides in mice. *Am. J. Respir. Crit. Care Med.* 2007;176(12):1243-1250.
[23] Zhou, S. F., Xue, C. C., Yu, X. Q., Li, C., Wang, G. Clinically important drug interactions potentially involving mechanism-based inhibition of cytochrome P450 3A4 and the role of therapeutic drug monitoring. *Ther. Drug Monit.* 2007;29(6):687-710.
[24] Dutreix, C., Peng, B., Mehring, G., et al. Pharmacokinetic interaction between ketoconazole and imatinib mesylate (Glivec) in healthy subjects. *Cancer Chemother. Pharmacol.* 2004;54(4):290-294.
[25] Foisy, M. M., Yakiwchuk, E. M., Huges, C. A. Induction effects of ritonavir: implications for drug interactions. *Ann. Pharmacother.* 2008; 42(7): 1048-1059.
[26] Haouala, A., Widmer, N., Duchosal, M. A., et al. Drug interactions with the tyrosine kinase inhibitors imatinib, dasatinib, and nilotinib. *Blood.* 2011 Feb. 24;117(8):e75-87.
[27] Kajita, T., Higashi, Y., Imamura, M., et al. Effect of imatinib mesilate on the disposition kinetics of ciclosporin in rats. *J. Pharm. Pharmacol.* 2006;58(7):997-1000.

[28] Frye, R. F., Fitzgerald, S. M., Lagattuta, T. F., Hruska, M. W., Egorin, M. J. Effect of St John's wort on imatinib mesylate pharmacokinetics. *Clin. Pharmacol. Ther.* 2004; 76(4):323-329.
[29] Smith, P., Bullock, J. M., Booker, B. M., et al. The influence of St. John's wort on the pharmacokinetics and protein binding of imatinib mesylate. *Pharma-cotherapy.* 2004; 24(11):1508-1514.
[30] Sparano, B. A., Egorin, M. J., Parise, R. A., et al. Effect of antacid on imatinib absorption. *Cancer Chemother. Pharmacol.* 2009;63(3):525-528.
[31] Ridruejo, E., Cacchione, R., Villamil, A. G., et al. Imatinib-induced fatal acute liver failure. *World J. Gastroenterol.* 2007;13(48):6608-111
[32] De Groot, J. W., Zonnenberg, B. A., Plukker, J. T., van Der Graaf, W. T., Links, T. P. Imatinib induces hypothyroidism in patients receiving levothyroxine. *Clin. Pharmacol. Ther.* 2005;78(4):433-438.
[33] Capdeville, R., Buchdunger, E., Zimmermann, J., Matter, A. Glivec (STI571, imatinib), a rationally developed, targeted anticancer drug. *Nat. Rev. Drug Discov.* 2002;1(7):493-502.
[34] O' Brien, S. G., Guilhot, F., Larson, R. A., et al. IRIS Investigators. Imatinib compared with interferon and low-dose cytarabine for newly diagnosed chronic-phase chronic myeloid leukemia. *N Eng. J. Med.* 2003; 348(11): 994-1004.
[35] Druker, B. J., Guilhot, F., O'Brien, S. G., et al. IRIS Investigators. Five-year follow-up of patients receiving imatinib for chronic myeloid leukemia. *N Engl. J. Med.* 2006; 355 (23):2408-2417.
[36] Larson, R. A., Druker, B. J., Guilhot, F., et al. Imatinib pharmacokinetics and its correlation with response and safety in chronic-phase chronic myeloid leukemia: a subanalysis of the IRIS study. *Blood.* 2008;111:4022–4028.
[37] Brouard, M., Saurat, J. H. Cutaneous reactions to STI571. *N Engl. J. Med.* 2001;345: 618–619.
[38] Hsiao, L. T., Chung, H. M., Lin, J. T., et al. Stevens-Johnson syndrome after treatment with STI571: a case report. *Br. J. Haematol.* 2002;117:620–622.
[39] Kerkelä, R., Grazette, L., Yacobi, R., et al. Cardiotoxicity of the cancer therapeutic agent imatinib mesylate. *Nat. Med.* 2006 Aug.;12(8):908-16.
[40] Atallah, E., Kantarjian, H., Cortes, J. In reply to 'Cardiotoxicity of the cancer therapeutic agent imatinib mesylate'. *Nat. Med.* 2007 Jan; 13(1):14; author reply 15-6.
[41] Gambacorti-Passerini, C., Tornaghi, L., Franceschino, A., et al. In reply to 'Cardiotoxicity of the cancer therapeutic agent imatinib mesylate'. *Nat. Med.* 2007 Jan.; 13(1):13-4; author reply 15-6.
[42] Hatfield, A., Owen, S., Pilot, P. R. In reply to 'Cardiotoxicity of the cancer therapeutic agent imatinib mesylate' *Nat. Med.* 2007 Jan.; 13(1):13; author reply 15-6.
[43] Rosti, G., Martinelli, G., Baccarani, M. In reply to 'Cardiotoxicity of the cancer therapeutic agent imatinib mesylate'. *Nat. Med.* 2007 Jan.; 13(1):15; author reply 15-6.
[44] Estabragh, Z. R., Knight, K., Watmough, S. J., et al. A prospective evaluation of cardiac function in patients with chronic myeloid leukaemia treated with imatinib. *Leuk. Res.* 2011 Jan.;35(1):49-51. Epub. 2010 Oct 27.
[45] Berman, E., Nicolaides, M., Maki, R. G., et al. Altered bone and mineral metabolism in patients receiving imatinib mesylate. *N Engl. J. Med.* 2006;354:2006–2013. [PubMed]

[46] Liu, F., Malaval, L., Aubin, J. E. Global amplification polymerase chain reaction reveals novel transitional stages during osteoprogenitor differentiation. *J. Cell Sci.* 2003;116:1787–1796.

[47] Tibullo, D., Giallongo, C., La Cava, P., et al. Effects of imatinib mesylate in osteoblastogenesis. *Exp. Hematol.* 2009;37:461–468

[48] Fitter, S., Dewar, A. L., Kostakis, P., et al. Long-term imatinib therapy promotes bone formation in CML patients. *Blood.* 2008;111:2538–2547.

[49] Grey, A., O'Sullivan, S., Reid, I. R., Browett, P. Imatinib mesylate, increased bone formation, and secondary hyperparathyroidism. *N Engl. J. Med.* 2006;355:2494–2495.

[50] O'Sullivan, S., Horne, A., Wattie, D., et al. Decreased bone turnover despite persistent secondary hyperparathyroidism during prolonged treatment with imatinib. *J. Clin. Endocrinol. Metab.* 2009;94:1131–1136.

[51] Hock, J. M., Canalis, E. Platelet-derived growth factor enhances bone cell replication, but not differentiated function of osteoblasts. *Endocrinology.* 1994;134:1423–1428.

[52] Fiedler, J., Etzel, N., Brenner, R. E. To go or not to go: migration of human mesenchymal progenitor cells stimulated by isoforms of PDGF. *J. Cell Biochem.* 2004; 93:990–998.

[53] Frédéric, M., Baruchel, A., Guilhot, J., et al. Imatinib is efficient but has a negative impact on growth in children with previously untreated chronic myelogenous leukemia (CNL) in early chronic phase (CP): results of the French National Phase IV trial. *ASH proceedings; 2009;* [Abstract 863].

[54] Pye, S. M., Cortes, J., Ault, P., et al. The effects of imatinib on pregnancy outcome. *Blood.* 2008 Jun. 15;111(12):5505-8.

[55] Ault, P., Kantarjian, H., O'Brien, S., et al. Pregnancy among patients with chronic myeloid leukemia treated with imatinib. *J. Clin. Oncol.* 2006 Mar. 1;24(7):1204-8.

[56] Kuwabara, A., Babb, A., Ibrahim, A., et al. Poor outcome after reintroduction of imatinib in patients with chronic myeloid leukemia who interrupt therapy on account of pregnancy without having achieved an optimal response. *Blood.* 2010 Aug. 12;116(6): 1014-6.

[57] Mughal, T. I., Schrieber, A. Principal long-term adverse effects of imatinib in patients with chronic myeloid leukemia in chronic phase. *Biologics.* 2010 Dec. 2;4:315-23

[58] Capdeville, R., Krahnke, T., Hatfield, A., Ford et al. Report of an international expanded access program of imatinib in adults with Philadelphia chromosome positive leukemias. *Ann. Oncol.* 2008 Jul.;19(7):1320-6.

In: Imatinib
Editors: Mojtaba Akhtari and Ihab Elhemaidi
ISBN: 978-1-62808-297-5

Chapter 2

Clinical Pharmacokinetics of Imatinib and Its Therapeutic Relevance

Nicolas Widmer,* Verena Gotta, Amina Haouala, Jaurès Blanc, Margaret von Mehren, Michel A. Duchosal, Serge Leyvraz, Chantal Csajka, Laurent A. Decosterd and Thierry Buclin

Division of Clinical Pharmacology, Service of Biomedicine,
Service and Central Laboratory of Hematology, Multidisciplinary Oncology Center;
Centre Hospitalier Universitaire Vaudois and University of Lausanne, Lausanne, Switzerland
Department of Medical Oncology, Fox Chase Cancer Center,
Philadelphia, Pennsylvania, USA
School of Pharmaceutical Sciences,
University of Geneva and University of Lausanne, Geneva, Switzerland

Abstract

The pharmacokinetic profile of imatinib has been assessed in healthy subjects and in population studies among thousands of patients with CML or GIST. Imatinib is rapidly and extensively absorbed from the GI tract, reaching a peak plasma concentration (C_{max}) within 1–4 h following administration. Imatinib bioavailability is high (98%) and independent of food intake. Imatinib undergoes rapid and extensive distribution into tissues, with minimal penetration into the central nervous system. In the circulation, it is approximately 95% bound to plasma proteins, principally α1-acid glycoprotein (AGP) and albumin. Imatinib undergoes metabolism in the liver via the cytochrome P_{450} enzyme system (CYP), with CYP3A4 being the main isoenzyme involved. The N-desmethyl

* Corresponding author: Nicolas Widmer. Division of Clinical Pharmacology, Centre Hospitalier Universitaire Vaudois and University of Lausanne, Hôpital de Beaumont 06.605, 1011 Lausanne, Switzerland. Phone:+41 21 314 42 69; Fax: +41 21 314 42 66; E-mail: Nicolas.Widmer@chuv.ch.

metabolite CGP74588 is the major circulating active metabolite. The typical elimination half-life for imatinib is approximately 14-22 h. Imatinib is characterized by large inter-individual pharmacokinetic variability, which reflects in a wide spread of concentrations observed under standard dosage. Besides adherence, several factors have been shown to influence this variability, especially demographic characteristics (sex, age, body weight and disease diagnosis), blood count characteristics, enzyme activity (mainly CYP3A4), drug interactions, activity of efflux transporters and plasma levels of AGP.

Additionally, recent retrospective studies have shown that drug exposure, reflected in either the area under the concentration-time curve (AUC) or more conveniently the trough level (C_{min}), correlates with treatment outcomes. Increased toxicity has been associated with high plasma levels, and impaired clinical efficacy with low plasma levels. While no upper concentration limit has been formally established, a lower limit for imatinib C_{min} of about 1000 ng/mL has been proposed repeatedly for improving outcomes in CML and GIST patients.

Imatinib is licensed for use in chronic phase CML and GIST at a fixed dose of 400 mg once daily (600 mg in some other indications) despite substantial pharmacokinetic variability caused by both genetic and acquired factors. The dose can be modified on an individual basis in cases of insufficient response or substantial toxic effects. Imatinib would, however, meet traditional criteria for a therapeutic drug monitoring (TDM) program: long-term therapy, measurability, high inter-individual but restricted intra-individual variability, limited pharmacokinetic predictability, effect of drug interactions, consistent association between concentration and response, suggested therapeutic threshold, reversibility of effect and absence of early markers of efficacy and toxic effects. Large-scale, evidence-based assessments of drug concentration monitoring are therefore still warranted for the personalization of imatinib treatment.

Introduction

The introduction of imatinib mesylate (Glivec®, Gleevec®; Novartis Pharma, Basel, Switzerland) represented an unprecedented clinical step forward in the management of patients with chronic myeloid leukemia (CML) and advanced gastrointestinal stromal tumors (GIST). Imatinib, arguably the archetype for tyrosine kinase inhibitors (TKI) [1], has produced outstanding long-term remissions during all clinical trials performed to confirm its effectiveness in these two malignancies [2-6]. However, failure to achieve the best possible clinical outcome is observed in a fraction of individual patients, and maximizing the long-term clinical benefits from imatinib may still require dose optimization and strategies to ensure proper adherence to therapy. Circulating drug concentrations appear to be correlated with outcomes in CML [7-20] and GIST patients [21-23]. Understanding the pharmacokinetic behavior of imatinib and controlling its circulating or intracellular concentration might therefore be crucial to optimize this oral maintenance treatment in patients receiving it [24, 25].

The pharmacokinetic (PK) profile of imatinib has been assessed among dozens of healthy subjects and thousands of CML and GIST patients [2, 3, 6, 7, 24, 26-28]. Moreover, several population pharmacokinetic (PopPK) analyses have been performed to investigate the variability of concentration exposure among different patient populations and to identify influential covariates [21, 23, 29-35]. The typical PK curve that can be derived from these PopPK is presented in Figure 1 [35].

Clinical Pharmacokinetic Profile

Absorption

Imatinib is rapidly and extensively absorbed from the gastro-intestinal tract, usually reaching a peak plasma concentration (C_{max}) within 1-4 h following administration [27, 28, 36]. The median duration of absorption (D1) is estimated to be 1.0 – 3.3 h [35]. Imatinib absorption is independent of food intake [37, 38] and its mean absolute bioavailability was estimated at about 98% [26, 27]. Presently marketed film-coated 100-mg and 400-mg tablet dose forms of imatinib are bioequivalent to the 100-mg hard-gelatin capsule initially commercialized [39]. Solid data on the bioequivalence of new imatinib generic formulations remains to be published.

Concomitant administration of Mg^{2+}-Al^{3+}–based antacids or proton pump inhibitors is not associated with meaningful alterations in imatinib absorption [40, 41]. In GIST patients, imatinib trough level (C_{min}) was significantly lower in patients with major gastrectomy than without (942 ± 330 ng/mL *versus* 1’393 ± 659 ng/mL, respectively; p=0.002). Such surgery appears therefore to impair imatinib absorption, possibly because of decreased transit time in the gastrointestinal system or lack of gastric acid secretion [42].

Distribution

Imatinib undergoes rapid and extensive distribution into body tissues [27]. The median apparent volume of distribution (Vd/F) ranges from 168 to 430 L [7, 35]. In the circulation, it is highly bound to plasma proteins (up to about 95%) [32, 36, 41, 43, 44] and to blood cells (8-30%) [27, 44]. Moreover, various uptake and efflux drug transporters mediate transport into and out of cells.

Binding studies of imatinib in plasma, in particular to human serum albumin (HSA) and α1-acid glycoprotein (AGP), showed a strong affinity for AGP, resulting in a mean free fraction of about 4% [32, 44]. An *in vitro* binding study with radioactive imatinib incubated in physiological conditions reported free fractions of 3.1% and 20% in AGP and HSA solutions, respectively, and of 4.3% in healthy human plasma [44]. Several studies showed that imatinib has about 50 to 60-fold higher affinity for AGP than for HSA [45, 46]. AGP in most individuals is a mixture of two or three genetic variants (F1 and/or S and A), which are encoded by two different genes [47, 48]. The F1 and S forms are encoded by alleles of the same gene, while the A variant is the product of the other gene. Imatinib binds with a stronger selectivity to the F1-S genetic variant of AGP, while its binding to the A variant is weaker and less specific [47, 48].

Imatinib has also been shown to be a substrate of the uptake drug transporter SLC22A1 (human organic cation transporter 1; hOCT1), as well as of the efflux transporters ABCB1 (P-glycoprotein; P-gp), and ABCG2 (breast cancer resistance protein; BCRP) [49-53]. However, a controversial report [54] has suggested that imatinib is an inhibitor rather than a substrate of BCRP, thus leaving uncertainty about the actual role of this transporter (see “cellular pharmacokinetics” section below).

Of importance, imatinib has been reported to only marginally cross the blood-brain barrier. This could be related to the high levels of P-gp in this barrier [55], as suggested by the increased brain penetration of imatinib after the administration of the P-gp inhibitor pantoprazole [56]. A low brain penetration was found to influence the therapeutic response of a CML patient who unexpectedly experienced a blastic crisis affecting the CNS, although having achieved complete cytological remission in his bone marrow. The levels of imatinib and of its active metabolite in this patient were 40-fold lower in the cerebrospinal fluid than in plasma [57]. In 17 patients the average CSF/plasma ratio was 1.8%, with an inter-individual variability (coefficient of variation, CV) of 71% [55].

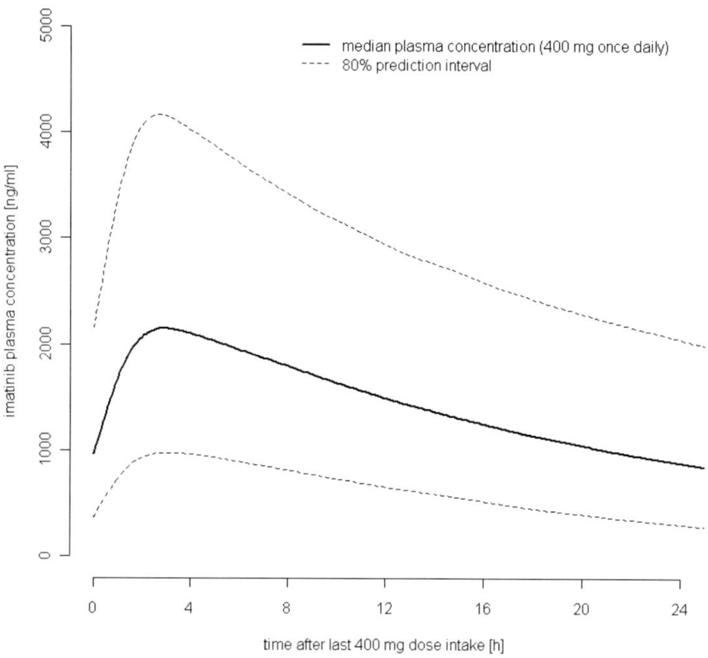

Figure 1. Typical pharmacokinetic profile of imatinib after a standardized 400 mg dose intake (dashed lines = 10th and 90th percentile, respectively). This simulation is based on a systematic review of PopPK analyses published to date [35].

Elimination

Only a negligible fraction of parent imatinib is found unchanged in urine [28, 58]. The drug undergoes extensive metabolism in the liver through the cytochrome P_{450} enzyme system (CYP), with CYP3A4 being the main isoenzyme involved [27, 36]. The drug is also metabolized, to a minor extent, by the CYP isoenzymes 1A2, 2C9 and 2C19, 2D6 and 3A5 [27, 59]. The fecal-to-urinary excretion ratio is about 5:1 [28]. On the other hand, imatinib is only a moderate inhibitor of CYP2C9, 2C19, 2D6 and 3A4 [60, 61] while its main metabolite is an inhibitor of CYP2D6 [36]. Imatinib median half-life (95% confidence interval) is estimated to range from 14 to 22 h [35]. The N-desmethyl metabolite CGP74588 is the major circulating active metabolite [27, 62, 63]. Its *in vitro* potency is similar to imatinib and its half-life is about 20 to 40 h. It represents however no more than 10% of the circulating amount of active drug [27, 28, 36] after a single oral dose, and no more than 20% at steady state [55].

Imatinib mean systemic clearance (CL/F) ranges between 9 and 14 L/h [35, 58]. This represents 19-31% of the normal liver plasma flow rate [7, 65] which indicates a rather low hepatic extraction ratio. As imatinib is highly bound to plasma proteins and blood cells, the determinant factors for its elimination are thus the intrinsic hepatic clearance and free fraction [35].

In liver dysfunction patients, somewhat surprisingly, no relationship was observed between imatinib PK and the severity of dysfunction [66, 67].

Finally and unexpectedly, a progressive increase in imatinib exposure with worsening renal function was observed, possibly because of altered plasma protein levels or anemia (low count of blood cells that bind imatinib) [67, 68]. No dose modifications are required for patients with mild or moderate renal dysfunction, but in patients with severe dysfunction, caution is advised owing to a lack of data [67, 68].

Pharmacokinetic Variability

Imatinib is characterized by large inter-individual pharmacokinetic variability, which is reflected in a wide range of concentrations observed under the standard dosage of 400 mg once daily, extending from 150 to more than 4000 ng/mL at the end of the dosage interval (C_{min}) [35]. The interquartile range (IQR) and median drug exposure, derived from simulations based on eight pooled PopPK models [21, 23, 29-34], were respectively 520-1390 ng/mL (grand median: 870 ng/mL) for C_{min} and 29-48 mg/L·h (grand median: 37 mg/L·h) for the area under the concentration-time curve (AUC) [35]. Table 1 summarizes the main PK parameters of imatinib [35].

The largest variability is attributed to absorption rate constant (total CV: 75-93%, estimated in 4 PopPK models) [21, 32-34], followed by Vd/F (total CV: 31-63%) [21, 23, 29-31, 34] and CL/F (total CV: 19-55%) [21, 23, 29-34]. A marked heterogeneity between studies is however observed [35]. Proportional residual intra-individual variability ranged from 22% to 40%, lower than the inter-individual variability [21, 23, 29-34].

Besides drug-drug interactions and adherence issues, addressed in the following sections of this chapter, several factors have been shown to explain some part of this variability, namely demographic characteristics (body weight [BW], sex, age, and disease diagnosis), plasma protein levels (AGP and HSA), blood count characteristics (granulocyte [GC] or white blood cell [WBC] count and hemoglobin [Hb] level), and duration of imatinib treatment (day 1 *versus* ≥1 month) [21, 23, 29-35]. A possible influence of a polymorphism affecting ABCG2 was found as well but need to be confirmed [32].

Besides age and disease diagnosis that affected only CL/F, most of the examined covariates influenced both CL/F and V/F to a similar extent. The effect was marked for BW (up to 50-70% increase in CL/F and V/F with doubling BW to 105 kg), albumin (up to 50% decrease in CL/F and V/F with hypoalbuminemia at 30 g/L), AGP (up to 50% increase in CL/F and 80% increase in V/F for low levels at 0.5 g/l), WBC (up to 80% increase in CL/F and V/F in case of leuco- or neutropenia below 2 G/L) and Hb (up to 35% decrease in CL/F and V/F for moderate anemia below 9 g/L) [35].

The effect of duration under imatinib treatment was not consistent between these retrospective studies, when comparing day 1 with "steady state" (day 29 or 12 months) CL/F or V/F estimates [35]. A recent prospective PopPK analysis has however observed a significant decrease in imatinib systemic exposure of 29.3% compared to baseline ($p<0.01$) [69]. Variations in AGP plasma levels might however have represented a confounding factor.

Table 1. Typical pharmacokinetic parameters of imatinib, derived from a systematic review of PopPK analyses published to date [35]

Parameter	Median value (IC95%)	Median value [IQR]
D1 [h]	1.7 (1.3 - 2.0)	
CL/F [L/h]	10.8 (9.3 - 12.4)	
V/F [L]	271.8 (214.2 - 329.3)	
AUC [mg/L·h]		37 [29 - 48]
C_{min} [ng/mL]		870 [530 -1390]

IC95%: 95% confidence interval of summary median, calculated by random-effect meta-analysis of reported medians and standard errors [35]. IQR: interquartile range, calculated on simulated concentrations from 9 population pharmacokinetic model [35].

Pharmacokinetic-Pharmacodynamic Relationships

As previously mentioned, retrospective studies have shown that drug exposure, reflected in either the AUC or more conveniently C_{min} (considered as either a threshold level *per se* or as a surrogate for AUC), correlated with treatment outcomes in both CML [7-20] and GIST patients [21-23].

Increased toxicity was associated with higher plasma levels, and impaired clinical efficacy with lower plasma levels. While no upper concentration limit has been formally established, a lower limit for imatinib C_{min} has been proposed repeatedly for improving outcomes in CML and GIST patients, namely 1000 and 1100 ng/mL, respectively [8]. These cut-offs have however been debated in the light of some controversial results. A few studies did not find a correlation with treatment response [21, 22, 29, 70-72], which can probably be attributed to observational and retrospective study designs [22, 70], short follow-up [21], limited patient numbers and selection biases [29, 71-73].

In addition, average exposures reported in responders and non-responders are rather heterogeneous and difficult to compare, because of differences in dosage regimens and patient characteristics (e.g. age, ethnicity) [18, 72].

Moreover, the response to treatment could also depend of various mutation profiles affecting the drug target in CML and GIST (BCR-ABL [74, 75] and KIT/PDFGR [76], respectively).

Correlating Imatinib Exposure with Response in CML

Among patients with CML, significant correlations between imatinib C_{min} and response have been found repeatedly [6, 77].

According to simulations from PK-PD models established during a phase I study (n=64) [7], the 1-month complete hematological response (CHR) rate is estimated at approximately 55%, 72% and 85% under imatinib C_{min} of 500, 700 or 1000 ng/mL (or AUC of 20, 30 or 45 mg/L·h) [35].

In a case-control study under fixed dosage (400 mg/day) [10], responders (CHR at 3 months or at least partial cytogenetic response [PCyR] at 6 months, n=20) had a median C_{min} of 952 ng/mL *versus* 302 ng/mL in non-responders (n=20; p=0.002) [35].

A lower threshold of 560 ng/mL [16] was estimated for optimal response by receiver operating characteristics (ROC; $AUC_{ROC\text{-}curve}$: 0.78), close to the concentration reported to inhibit proliferation of Ph+ leukemic cells obtained from patients with CML by 60-80% (1 μM ≈ 570 ng/mL [35, 78]).

Several reports have investigated the rate of complete cytogenetic response (CCyR; no more Ph+ cells detectable) or major molecular response (MMR; ≥ 3-log reduction from baseline in abnormal BCR-ABL mRNA transcript level or ≤ 0.1% on the international scale) [35], mainly including patients receiving imatinib for more than 1 year – and up to 7 years [8, 12-15, 19, 20, 35, 70-72]. Fewer studies have provided estimates of early (6 to 18 months) cytogenetic response (CyR) or molecular response (MR) rates [9, 10, 12, 16-18, 35]. In a Korean study (n=87), optimal CyR at 6 months (PCyR or CCyR) was significantly lower in patients having C_{min} below 1000 ng/mL (80.6%) than in patients having C_{min} above 1000 ng/mL (94.6%, p=0.032) [17]. In the PK-PD subanalysis of the International Randomized Interferon *versus* STI571 (IRIS) trial data (n=351), patients with "low" C_{min} at day 29 (< 650 ng/mL, quartile Q1) had significantly lower cumulative CCyR (p=0.005) and MMR rates (p=0.008) than those with higher exposure [9]. Cumulative 1-year CCyR and MMR rates were 59% and 43% respectively, compared to 71-73% and 56-55% in patients with "average" (650-1180 ng/mL, Q2-Q3) to "high" exposure (> 1180 ng/mL, Q4). There was also a trend for a lower 5-year event-free survival (EFS) rate in the "low" versus "average" and "high" exposure groups (78% *versus* 83% and 89%; p=0.16). In the PK-PD analysis of the Tyrosine Kinase Dose Optimization Study (TOPS) trial [18] that included patients randomized 1:2 to 400 mg and 800 mg imatinib, C_{min} values were proportional to dose and stable over time despite high inter-patient variability. Patients with "low" imatinib C_{min} at day 28 (< 1165 ng/mL; Q1) had significantly lower 12-months CCyR/MMR rates (70%/38%) than patients with higher C_{min} (Q2-Q3: 86%/58%, p=0.01; Q4: 94%/59%, p=0.008). Optimal thresholds for improved response rates were proposed in 4 studies through ROC analysis: 560 ng/mL for optimal early CyR and HR (see above) [16]; 974 ng/mL [12] for 1-year MMR ($AUC_{ROC\text{-}curve}$ 0.74); and for overall MMR: 817 ng/mL (0.82) [12], 1002 ng/mL (0.78) [8] and 2158 ng/mL (0.85) [13], with the latter study reporting overall higher concentrations in the patients tested.

Finally, another analysis pooled data from patients with newly diagnosed and previously untreated Ph+ chronic phase CML from both the IRIS and TOPS trials. This study confirmed that higher steady-state imatinib levels correlated with better complete cytogenetic response (CCyR) and MMR, but also resulted in more grade 3 and 4 treatment-related toxicities [79].

Correlating Imatinib Exposure with Response in GIST

Consistent findings are also emerging from studies that examined the relationship between imatinib concentration exposure and response to treatment, as well as between free drug levels and side effects in GIST patients with imatinib [6].

In the PK-PD substudy of the US-Finish Phase II B2222 trial [23] that included 73 GIST patients randomized 1:1 to 400 mg or 600 mg, C_{min} was measured at day 29 and the best response (stable disease, partial or complete response; SD, PR or CR) during 5-years of follow-up was evaluated. 28 patients necessitated dosage increase because of disease progression during the study. Patients who had low C_{min} at day 29 (< 1110 ng/mL; Q1) had a lower rate of response (67%) and time to progression (11.3 months) than patients with higher C_{min} (67-74%, p=0.18, and 30 months, p=0.01, respectively), even though median overall survival did not differ (p=0.16). Another analysis [21] was performed on PK/PD data obtained during the French Phase III BFR14 trial [80] from 34 patients having started 400 mg imatinib without dosage modification. After 2 months, patients were assessed for treatment response with 44% having stable disease and 47% achieving a partial response; there was no difference in AUC between these two groups. In a Swiss analysis of observational PK/PD data from 38 GIST patients [22, 81], unbound imatinib exposure, rather than total exposure, was selectively associated with response in the subgroup of patients whose tumors harbored wild-type (WT) or exon 9 mutated KIT (see below).

Finally, preliminary French results (published in abstract form) showed that long-term survivors tended to have higher imatinib trough concentrations than more recently treated patients [82]. Additionally, the clinical database of the same group was analyzed to evaluate factors associated with longer progression free survival. This analysis of 102 patients treated with 400 mg/daily defined a C_{min} threshold of 780 ng/mL associated with 71% reduction of disease progression for advanced GIST arising from stomach or small bowel.

Altogether, these results in GIST patients appear rather heterogeneous, describing different concentration cut-offs. They may have been obscured by heterogeneity in patients' tumor genotypes, known to also influence clinical response (see next section). They certainly deserve further prospective investigations.

Correlating Imatinib Exposure and Response by Mutational Subtype

Imatinib response in GIST varies based on the type of activating mutation(s) present in tumor cells [4, 6, 83]. Mutational analysis of tumors from the large European Organisation for Research and Treatment of Cancer (EORTC)–Australasian Phase III trial, comparing response and survival following either standard-dose (400 mg daily) or high- dose (800 mg daily) imatinib, found that the presence of KIT exon 11 mutation was the strongest predictor of response and disease stabilization [76]. Tumors with KIT exon 9 mutation were associated with significantly poorer progression free survival (PFS) on standard-dose therapy, which was not observed in KIT exon 11 or WT tumors [76]. Similar results were reported from the North American Southwest Oncology Group (SWOG) S0033 Phase III trial, in which KIT exon 9 and WT genotypes predicted poorer response and shorter time to progression compared with KIT exon 11 mutations. There was some evidence of improved response in patients with exon 9 mutant genotype who received high-dose imatinib [84]. The Meta-GIST analysis of both

Phase III studies of imatinib indicated that imatinib 800 mg daily significantly improved PFS patients whose GIST harbored a KIT exon 9 mutation, in contrast to those that harbored other mutations [85].

In the B2222 PK-PD substudy, the presence of KIT exon 11 mutation predicted improved clinical benefit for imatinib exposure exceeding 1100 ng/mL [23]. In 39 patients with KIT exon 11 mutations evaluated for C_{min}, patients in the upper quartiles (Q2-Q4) had significantly higher rates of overall objective clinical response: 100% achieved either CR, PR, or SD compared with 67% for those in Q1 ($p=0.0001$) [23]. There were too few patients with KIT exon 9 mutations to draw firm conclusions among this subgroup.

Results from the Swiss analysis found the strongest association between free AUC and response among patients whose tumors harbored KIT exon 9 mutations or WT KIT [22].

In an additional analysis, the relationship between extrapolated free C_{min} and clinical response was shown to be especially relevant in patients whose tumors either contained a KIT exon 9 mutation or were WT [81]. Because of the limited number of patients included in the analysis, such results should be considered with caution and remain to be confirmed in further studies. In addition, using free imatinib levels derived from a per-sample analysis in these two studies may have led to an artificially over-powered analysis, as this approach ignores intra-patient correlation [22, 81]. Extrapolation of free concentrations also still remains to be confirmed formally by direct measurement of free plasma levels of imatinib in patients' blood (see "Free concentrations" section below).

Regarding imatinib response in CML, it could also depend of the various mutation profiles affecting the BCR-ABL drug target [74, 75]. However, no concentration-effect analyses have specifically addressed this question yet.

Correlating Imatinib Exposure with Adverse Events

In the above-cited IRIS trial, the imatinib discontinuation rate in CML patients due to adverse events (AEs) tended to be numerically higher in patients with "high" C_{min} (> 1180 ng/mL, Q4: 7%) than in patients with "average" (Q2-Q3: 2.8%) or "low" C_{min} (< 644 ng/mL, Q1: 4.6%, $p=0.28$), respectively [9, 35]. AEs more frequently reported in patients with high exposure were fluid retention (76% *versus* 62%, $p=0.027$, OR=1.9), skin rash (51% *versus* 39%; $p=0.064$, OR=1.7), anemia (20% *versus* 12%, $p=0.09$, OR=1.8) and nausea during the first 3 months (42% *versus* 27%, $p=0.02$, OR=1.9) [9]. In the TOPS trial, anemia was more frequent in CML patients with "high" drug exposure (C_{min} > 3180 ng/mL, Q4: 43%) than in patients with "average" (1165-3180 ng/mL, Q2-Q3: 24%; $p=0.01$) or "low" drug exposure (< 1165 ng/mL, Q1: 22%; $p=0.02$, OR=2.7) [18]. The only non-hematologic adverse event with a significant exposure relationship was skin rash (40% in Q4 *versus* 20% in Q1, $p=0.03$, OR=2.6) [18, 35].

Some subcategories of musculoskeletal adverse events, fluid retention and gastro-intestinal side effects also occurred more frequently in patients with high drug exposure, however they were not statistically significant [18, 35]. In the previously mentioned Swiss study, total AUC correlated with the number of side effects in GIST patients ($p<0.001$, OR: 2.2 for doubling AUC), even though unbound AUC was a better surrogate and predicted the number of side effects in CML patients [22].

In a French Phase III trial of imatinib in GIST patients [21] (n=32), total AUC correlated with hematotoxicity (neutropenia, thrombocyto-penia), even though to a lesser extent than unbound AUC (or AGP levels).

Notably, 6 out of 7 GIST patients with total AUC > 55 mg/L·h experienced a > 50% decrease in absolute neutrophil count. Interestingly, toxicity-adjusted low-dose imatinib seems to be effective in some CML [86, 87] and GIST [88] patients, even though no PK data in this context are available. This might however not apply to high-risk CML patients [89].

Free Concentrations

As mentioned above, recent results have demonstrated the importance of free drug concentrations of imatinib (i.e. the pharmacologically active fraction not bound to albumin or AGP) when considering exposure [6].

For drugs with low hepatic extraction and high protein binding such as imatinib, a change in protein concentrations or in binding affinity alters total plasma concentrations, while free drug levels are expected to remain mostly unchanged [65].

However, an altered free fraction modifies the apparent total concentration-effect relationships, and may thus compromise the correct interpretation of total plasma concentrations. Moreover, under certain pathophysiological conditions competing with normal binding, such as uremia, liver disease, hypoproteinemia or drug interactions, free drug concentration may be significantly elevated despite standard total concentrations [90].

The relationship between unbound drug exposure and efficacy and toxicity endpoints has been recently investigated (see previous section). These results were however obtained using extrapolated free concentrations rather than actual measurements. Their formal confirmation is therefore still warranted [41]. Some analytical methods devoted to the measurement of free drug levels have been recently published [41, 91, 92] and could be used to confirm the extrapolated data. Finally, it should be noted that a PopPK model was recently established using real free and total imatinib concentrations measurement to allow the confident prediction of imatinib free levels based on total concentrations and plasma AGP levels [41]. Free concentration measurement requires an additional ultrafiltration step and sensitive analytical technology, not widely available in clinical laboratories. This latter model might thus represent a convenient approach to estimate imatinib free levels with the following relationship [41]:

$$C_u = 0.5 \cdot \Big(C_{tot} - 319 - 11700 \cdot AGP_{tot} + \sqrt{(C_{tot} - 319 - 11700 \cdot AGP_{tot})^2 + 1276 \cdot C_{tot}}\Big)$$

where C_u and C_{tot} (imatinib free and total concentrations, respectively) are expressed in ng/mL and AGP_{tot} (AGP plasma levels) in g/L.

Cellular Pharmacokinetics

Up to now, investigations on PK/PD aspects of imatinib and other TKI therapies have focused almost exclusively on concentrations of the parent drug in plasma, considering it as the best pharmacokinetic marker predictive of clinical response (see previous sections). Nevertheless, the molecular target of imatinib in CML, BCR-ABL, resides within malignant cells. Moreover, for the GIST context, although the KIT/PDGFRA targets are located on the cell surface, the binding site of imatinib is intracellular as well. The drug cellular disposition, resulting from complex mutual biological, genetic and environmental influences, remains poorly described at present.

Therefore, a new research field addressing the so-called "cellular pharmacokinetics" is emerging, which aims at monitoring variables that would more closely reflect the intracellular environment of the therapeutic target, rather than the systemic blood concentrations currently measured.

The actual drug exposure within the cell can now be determined thanks to the capacity of highly sensitive mass spectrometry tools [93-95] and will certainly help at filling knowledge gaps in the PK-PD of TKIs, such as imatinib. It will thus allow understanding some instances of insufficient clinical response, resistance or intolerance to TKI treatment.

In a similar line of development, the subcellular distribution of imatinib is still largely unknown, a point that could be highly relevant considering that the target kinase is unevenly distributed in the leukemia cells cytoplasm (BCR-ABL) or that the binding site of imatinib is intracellular (KIT/PDGFRA).

Cellular Penetration in CML

As previously mentioned, the concentration of imatinib in the cell cytoplasm, although driven by circulating blood levels, is further dependent of various transmembrane transporters that mediate the inward (uptake) and outward (efflux) of drugs into leukemic cells. There is accumulating evidence indicating that variable expression of these drug transporters, and thus presumably variable intracellular concentration of imatinib, is a key determinant of response to treatment [96-99].

One study measured intracellular concentrations of imatinib in peripheral blood mononuclear cells (PBMC; used as a surrogate for target cells) from patients' peripheral blood samples [31]. Except for one subject, the intra-/extra-cellular ratio appeared rather constant, and indicated an average 8-fold accumulation of imatinib within cells as compared to plasma levels, in agreement with available *in vitro* data (approximate 5-fold factor in leukemia cell cultures incubated with imatinib and human plasma [55]). Such results were in line with the demonstration that imatinib undergoes active uptake into leukemia cells by hOCT1 [100]. There is evidence that hOCT1 represents a major contributor to clinical response in CML patients treated with imatinib [53, 100]. Functional activity of hOCT1 in mononuclear cells (MNC) collected from CML patients has indeed been related to molecular response to imatinib [96, 98, 99]. A relationship between hOCT1 mRNA levels and cytogenetic response rates to imatinib was also observed in other studies [101, 102]. However, while hOCT1 activity in mature MNC appears significantly associated with the achievement of MMR, no relationship was found between hOCT1 activity in CML CD34+ precursor cells and patients' molecular response rate [103].

Moreover, several studies provide evidence that imatinib is a substrate of P-gp, the archetypal member of the ABC transporter protein family [49, 93, 97, 104, 105]. For instance, striking differences (up to 24-fold) have been observed in intracellular concentrations of imatinib according to cells ability to express P-gp [50]. Imatinib was indeed very efficiently expelled from ABCB1+ cells at all tested concentrations. Several *in vitro* studies using pharmacological modulators or RNA interference (RNAi) knockdown of ABCB1 also suggest that ABCB1 activity can confer resistance to imatinib in CML K562 cell lines [49, 97, 106-108]. However, this has been questioned [109-111] and the clinical studies conducted so far have failed to correlate P-gp expression with resistance to imatinib [101, 112]. P-gp expression itself may therefore not represent a clinically relevant predictor of resistance in population studies.

Yet, protein expression levels may not correlate with functionality. Recently, three different single-nucleotide polymorphisms (SNP) in the ABCB1 gene were evaluated and correlated with MMR to imatinib therapy. Among patients homozygous for allele 1236T, 85% achieved a major molecular response *versus* 48% for the other genotypes (p=0.003) [113].

Finally, ABCG2 has also been implicated in the active efflux of imatinib from cells despite some initial controversial findings [114, 115].

The ultimate, although yet rarely achievable, goal of anticancer treatment is the eradication of tumor cells. In Ph+ leukemia, the critical determinant of the efficacy of imatinib therapy is the extent of BCR-ABL tyrosine kinase inhibition achieved, which depends on the concentration of TKIs in the cytoplasm environment.

However, all available studies on leukemic cell sensitivity to imatinib are based on imatinib concentrations in incubation medium, not in cells, which differ strikingly [93]. How imatinib concentration in the incubation medium confidently reflects cellular level and how it correlates with cancer cell responsiveness remains unknown at present. Thus information on actual imatinib concentration in the cytoplasm will be necessary for establishing accurate PK-PD relationships at the cellular level.

Imatinib Tissue Levels in GIST

No human PK data on imatinib tissue levels in GIST or other tissues where metastases disseminate is available at present [6]. Only one study has described the distribution of imatinib in small cell lung cancer xenografts in mice, showing that therapeutic concentrations of imatinib were achieved in plasma and tumor xenografts but not in the brain [116]. The liver distribution of imatinib has also been explored by tandem mass spectrometry in rats treated by imatinib for fibrogenesis. An inverse correlation of liver function and imatinib levels indicated that drug metabolism via CYP was impaired in fibrotic livers, resulting in higher drug-on-target levels in advanced fibrosis [117].

Drug Interactions

In line with the above-mentioned pharmacokinetic characteristics, various drug-drug interactions may influence the course of imatinib treatment [118].

Interactions should notably be considered when administering inhibitors of the CYP3A family in combination with imatinib. Strong CYP3A4 inhibition, such as achieved with ketoconazole, caused a 40% increase of imatinib exposure in healthy volunteers [119]. Interactions are also likely to occur with other inhibitors of CYP3A4, such as levothyroxine [120, 121], voriconazole [122], amiodarone [123] or even Ginseng [124], leading to an increase in plasma concentrations of imatinib. However, a study suggests that inhibition of CYP3A4 by the potent irreversible inhibitor ritonavir does not result in increased steady-state plasma concentrations of imatinib, possibly because of the induction of compensatory metabolism or transport mechanisms by ritonavir [125].

Administration of inhibitors of both CYP3A4 and P-gp with imatinib increases not only plasma but also intracellular imatinib concentrations. Dual CYP3A4 and P-gp inhibitors such as verapamil [126], erythromycin [127], clarithromycin [127], cyclosporine [128, 129], ketoconazole [119], fluconazole [118], itraconazole [118] and metronidazole [130] may increase intracellular concentrations of imatinib by inhibiting both its metabolism and its efflux by P-gp, and might therefore increase its cellular toxicity.

Interactions with quinidine, ranitidine or midazolam, known inhibitors of hOCT1, might paradoxically increase the circulating concentrations of imatinib but decrease the intracellular exposure of target cancer cells, known to express this carrier [53].

Concomitant administration of CYP3A4 inducers such as rifampicin or certain antiepileptics may lead to a reduction of as much as 74% in imatinib exposure [61, 131, 132]. Moreover, the pharmacokinetic profile of imatinib was significantly altered by St John's wort, with reductions of 30% in the median AUC [133, 134].

Data concerning interactions involving protein binding are poorly documented for imatinib. A study showed that St John's wort does not alter the protein binding of imatinib over a wide range of concentrations in vivo [134].

Imatinib can also inhibit drug transporters and enzymes, leading to changes in the circulating exposure to co-administered drugs. Imatinib enhances the intestinal absorption of cyclosporine, a CYP3A4 and P-gp substrate, and may increase its pharmacologic effects and possibly toxicity [128, 129].

Moreover, the clearance of simvastatin (a CYP3A4 substrate) was reduced by 70% when associated with imatinib [135]. Administration of imatinib together with metoprolol, a CYP2D6 substrate, resulted in an increase in metoprolol exposure by 23% [136]. Additionally, imatinib is also known to inhibit the O-glucuronidation of acetaminophen, possibly inducing hepatotoxicity and liver failure following the intake of high doses [118]. The use of acetaminophen should therefore be limited to 1300 mg per day in patients taking imatinib, despite some recent controversies [137, 138]. Monitoring liver function tests during prolonged treatment is useful [139]. Acenocoumarol and phenprocoumon, substrates of CYP 2C9, show also increased concentrations; however, a clinically dangerous interaction can be prevented by the monitoring of prothrombin time or international normalized ratio [118].

Physicians should also be aware that patients with hypothyroid conditions who receive imatinib need increased levothyroxine dosages [120, 121]. The suspected mechanism is an induction of non–deiodination clearance. A 2-fold increase in levothyroxine substitution therapy at initiation of imatinib treatment is therefore recommended, along with close monitoring of thyroid function [120, 121].

With regard to all these mechanisms, it is worth to remember that plasma concentrations of imatinib are correlated with both efficacy and toxicity [7-23]. A change in imatinib exposure due to drug interactions might therefore definitely influence its therapeutic efficacy, and has been actually found in a large European observational study to be published.

Impact of Adherence

Oral cancer therapies, such as imatinib, have become increasingly common in oncology practice [6, 25]. Although they offer patients the convenience of self-administration at home, evidence suggests that adherence to oral cancer therapies is far from optimal [140-143]. A number of recent studies have examined adherence to imatinib therapy among patient populations with either GIST or CML; all documented surprisingly high rates of non-adherence [141, 142, 144].

In one study, patient prescription data were collected among 4043 patients receiving imatinib for CML or GIST for 24 months [142]. The overall rate of compliance (doses of imatinib taken *versus* dosage prescribed) for both patient groups was 75%. Total (100%) compliance was achieved by only half of the patients. During the course of the 24-month study, average persistence was 255 days (time that each patient remained on therapy). As seen in other disease categories, a high and stable level of persistence was observed early in the treatment course, followed by a steady decline [142]. Another study examined prescription data in 320 patients, who received imatinib therapy for CML or GIST during a period of 12 months. The average rate of full compliance was 76%. More than a quarter of patients (28%) interrupted therapy for at least 30 consecutive days [141]. Factors associated with non-adherence in this study included increasing age (older than 51 years), gender (female), higher number of concomitant medications, and complications of disease or therapy [141]. The Adherence Assessment with Glivec®: Indicators and Outcomes (ADAGIO) study was an observational, open-label trial conducted in 169 patients with chronic phase CML who received imatinib [144]. Approximately one-third of included patients exhibited non-adherent behavior. Patterns of under- and overtaking medication were evident using pill-count data, with perfect adherence reported in only 14.2% of patients. Factors associated with non-adherence to imatinib therapy included increased age, increased time since diagnosis, being male (in contrast with the previous study), increased duration of imatinib treatment, and improved health at study [144].

Because imatinib therapy requires daily administration, maintaining proper adherence is essential to obtain a stable pharmacokinetic profile of the drug. This may be of greater significance in patients with advanced GIST, as discontinuation of imatinib is associated with loss of remission and a shorter time to progression, even in patients who have achieved complete response when imatinib is discontinued [6]. This is supported by the Phase III French Sarcoma Group BFR14 Study evaluating the effect of imatinib interruption in responding patients after different periods of treatment [80, 145]. One-, 3- and 5-year results from the study indicate that discontinuation of imatinib is associated with rapid progression

[80, 145]. Conversely, in CML, early studies showed that discontinuation of imatinib might be feasible after sustained complete molecular response has been achieved (41% of probability of persistent complete molecular response at 12 month) [146]. Moreover, in patients relapsing, previous best responses can be achieved following imatinib re-introduction [146, 147]. However, in another study, prolonged dose interruptions in CML patients compromise CCyR and MMR rates at 12 months [79]. Nevertheless, continuous administration is probably appropriate for most patients.

Therapeutic Drug Monitoring

Therapeutic drug monitoring (TDM) to achieve defined circulating drug concentrations by adjusting dosage regimens is not commonly used in oncology at present [6]. However, it is employed in several other medical disciplines, including organ transplant, cardiology, neurology, and infectious disease (including HIV/AIDS, a disease with pharmacotherapeutic requirements that roughly resemble GIST and CML) [6, 148]. Procedures to monitor treatment continue to be developed, mainly based on empirical practice rather than on robust evidence. Worldwide, these procedures receive insufficient consideration from researchers, and appropriate research methodologies still need to be refined [148, 149].

In a competitive economic framework, pharmaceutical companies are reluctant to encourage approaches that might complicate the prescription of their drugs. In parallel, public funders show little interest in supporting trials to improve the use of products that generate private profits [150]. This context results in a substantial lack of incentives to optimize use of long-term therapies, such as TKIs. However, it is not the administered dose but the systemic concentration that drives the efficacy and toxic effects of most drugs.

Imatinib is licensed for use in chronic phase CML and GIST at a fixed dose of 400 mg once daily (600 mg in some indications) despite substantial pharmacokinetic variability caused by both genetic and acquired factors (see previous sections). The dose can be modified on an individual basis in cases of insufficient response or substantial toxic effects. As previously suggested, imatinib would however meet traditional criteria for a therapeutic drug monitoring program: long-term therapy; measurability; high inter-individual but restricted intra-individual variability; limited pharmacokinetic predictability; effect of drug interactions; consistent associations between concentration and response; suggested therapeutic threshold; reversibility of effect; and absence of early efficacy or markers of toxic effects [150, 151]. TDM for imatinib may therefore provide additional information on efficacy, compliance, and safety compared to clinical evaluation alone [151]. Moreover, in CML, it could be hypothesized that TDM could contribute to achieve faster a complete molecular response (CMR) that might be a prerequisite for a possible cure of the disease [146]. As mentioned above, findings from recent studies have improved our understanding of the relationship between imatinib exposure and clinical outcomes, but the putative plasma threshold for clinical benefit remains a subject of investigation [6]. Moreover, no prospective clinical trial has assessed the use of imatinib TDM to date [150]. Suitable blood levels needs especially to be prospectively evaluated in various patient subgroups (in term of minimal as well as maximal levels). To that purpose, in CML, a randomized controlled trial (Imatinib COncentration Monitoring Evaluation; I-COME) is ongoing in Switzerland [152]. For GIST, the Sarcoma Alliance for Research through Collaboration (SARC) Imatinib TDM Study (SARC-019) might have provide important answers in US patients, but has been terminated due to very slow accrual [153].

In the current stage of knowledge, applications for TDM during imatinib therapy might include suboptimal or possibly lack of therapeutic response, severe or unexpected toxicities, drug–drug interactions, and monitoring of adherence to treatment [6, 77, 151, 154, 155]. Moreover, evidence suggests that dose adjustment based on TDM might be beneficial for most TKIs, not just for imatinib [25, 156]. Individualization of TKIs dosage by TDM could represent the next step towards a further refinement for targeted anticancer therapies, aiming at administering "the right dose of the right drug to the right patient". In this emerging field of personalized medicine, the development of TDM for patient-tailored dose adjustment should maximize both the therapeutic benefit and the tolerability of these new drugs [151].

Practical Issues

The currently preferred analytical method for imatinib TDM is liquid chromatography–tandem mass spectrometry (LC-MS/MS) [95]. It provides a rapid, efficient, and simple means of quantifying imatinib in plasma. The method has been shown to be precise, sensitive, and accurate. LC-MS/MS assays are presently being developed to cover other major TKIs [94, 157, 158]. Although LC-MS/MS is the preferred method for imatinib TDM, cost considerations may prohibit its use in certain settings [6]. High-performance liquid chromatography–ultraviolet (HPLC-UV) techniques have also been published, making the assay accessible by any laboratory or institute not equipped with sophisticated and costly LC-MS/MS apparatus [159, 160].

Major cancer treatment centers in Europe, in collaboration with the manufacturer of imatinib, have developed a testing protocol for monitoring plasma levels in cancer patients under the frame of the European Treatment and Outcome Study (EUTOS) of the European Leukemia Net [161]. This effort is focused on developing a database of imatinib plasma level measurements to verify therapeutic plasma thresholds in various indications and to identify and certify laboratories to provide proper testing services [6]. Initially, an external quality control program had been organized at the Bordeaux University Hospital (France). Some private laboratories currently provide external quality control samples for imatinib and some other TKIs [95].

In clinical practice, the development of mathematical algorithms, such as Bayesian approach, will enable the drawing of samples at time points not strictly corresponding to the trough level, thus, providing a wider sampling window [162, 163]. However, current recommendations for imatinib sampling are still 24 h post-dose for the imatinib 400 mg daily dosing and 12 h post-dose for the imatinib 400 mg twice-daily dosing. Moreover, because of some observations suggesting modifications of imatinib exposure over time [29, 69], TDM could also be time-point specific [164].

The monitoring of imatinib is currently based on total concentrations of imatinib. However, as above-mentioned, considering either the free concentrations or the cellular concentration of the drug might be more relevant (Figure 2). Such concentrations thresholds are unknown yet, but some analytical techniques are being developed to measure unbound [91, 92] or intracellular [93, 165] imatinib concentrations.

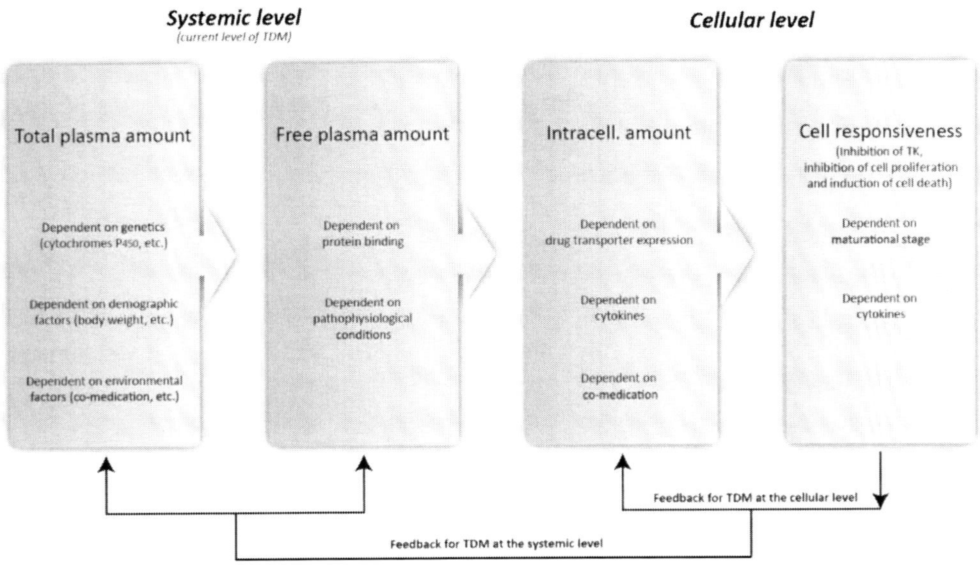

Figure 2. Levels of interest of PK-PD relationships.

These measurement techniques could be used to investigate further free and cellular concentration-effect relationships, as well as the associated TDM approach. As previously discussed, extrapolating free imatinib concentration based on imatinib total and AGP plasma concentrations could also be advised [41].

Finally, concerning the issue of treatment compliance, it is worth noting that a French study observed in four of seven patients very low trough levels resulting from poor adherence [82]. Although TDM may be useful in this context, it is important to recall that measured drug levels are only indicative of short-term compliance and may not reflect adherence during any prolonged period prior to testing. Also, TDM may indeed be subject to a confounding "white coat" effect when used to assess adherence [166].

Conclusion

Long-term studies of imatinib have documented impressive rates of response and survival. Moreover, the pharmacokinetics of the drug has been extensively studied and well documented, as shown in the review. Nevertheless, achieving optimal clinical benefit from imatinib depends on optimal concentration exposure, which can be affected by factors such as individual patient variability in absorption, distribution, and metabolism, due to genetic or demographic differences, anatomical or post-surgery anomalies of the GI tract. Other specific factors, such as adherence, drug interactions or environmental influences may also impact on drug exposure, thus potentially compromising adequate response [6].

New therapeutic agents such as imatinib are revolutionizing cancer treatment, and some of them have transformed deadly malignancies into chronically manageable conditions. Nevertheless, primary or secondary drug resistance, persistence of cancer stem cells, and adverse drug effects still limit their ability to stabilize or even cure malignant diseases in the long term [95].

In addition, poor tolerance and therapeutic failure are not uncommon, and relapse is a nearly inevitable consequence of treatment interruption. The appropriate management of oncologic patients therefore requires careful monitoring of these novel treatments [75, 167], for which most clinicians have still a rather limited experience. For imatinib, it appears that this can be done through the TDM approach, whereby the careful selection of drug dosage is adapted to each patient according to individual plasma concentrations. This will minimize the risk of major adverse reactions and to increase the probability of efficient, long-lasting, therapeutic response [151].

The outcomes of randomized prospective trials testing the clinical benefits of TDM are however still eagerly awaited by clinicians to define the exact role of TDM in imatinib treatment personalization [6, 150, 151].

Acknowledgments

The development and application of imatinib blood measurement at the Division of Clinical Pharmacology (Centre Hospitalier Universitaire Vaudois and University of Lausanne, Switzerland) has benefited from an unrestricted grant from Novartis Pharma Schweiz (Bern, Switzerland), especially through the I-COME study.

The present review work was also partly supported by the Swiss National Science Foundation (Bern, Switzerland) through the "Intelligent Integrated Systems for Personalized Medicine" (ISyPeM; Nano-Tera Initiative, grant no. 128852) and "Integrative cellular pharmacokinetics-pharmacodynamics-pharmacoproteomics studies of anticancer tyrosine kinase inhibitors in leukemia" projects (grant no. 138097).

References

[1] Sawyers, C. Targeted cancer therapy. *Nature* 2004; 432(7015): 294-7.

[2] Druker, B. J., Talpaz, M., et al. Efficacy and safety of a specific inhibitor of the BCR-ABL tyrosine kinase in chronic myeloid leukemia. *N Engl. J. Med.* 2001; 344(14): 1031-7.

[3] Demetri, G. D., von Mehren, M., et al. Efficacy and safety of imatinib mesylate in advanced gastrointestinal stromal tumors. *N Engl. J. Med.* 2002; 347(7): 472-80.

[4] Blanke, C. D., Demetri, G. D., et al. Long-term results from a randomized phase II trial of standard- versus higher-dose imatinib mesylate for patients with unresectable or metastatic gastrointestinal stromal tumors expressing KIT. *J. Clin. Oncol.* 2008; 26(4): 620-5.

[5] Hochhaus, A., Druker, B., et al. Favorable long-term follow-up results over 6 years for response, survival, and safety with imatinib mesylate therapy in chronic-phase chronic myeloid leukemia after failure of interferon-alpha treatment. *Blood* 2008; 111(3): 1039-43.

[6] von Mehren, M., Widmer, N. Correlations between imatinib pharmacokinetics, pharmacodynamics, adherence, and clinical response in advanced metastatic

gastrointestinal stromal tumor (GIST): an emerging role for drug blood level testing? *Cancer Treat. Rev.* 2011; 37(4): 291-9.

[7] Peng, B., Hayes, M., et al. Pharmacokinetics and pharmacodynamics of imatinib in a phase I trial with chronic myeloid leukemia patients. *J. Clin. Oncol.* 2004; 22(5): 935-42.

[8] Picard, S., Titier, K., et al. Trough imatinib plasma levels are associated with both cytogenetic and molecular responses to standard-dose imatinib in chronic myeloid leukemia. *Blood* 2007; 109(8): 3496-9.

[9] Larson, R. A., Druker, B. J., et al. Imatinib pharmacokinetics and its correlation with response and safety in chronic phase chronic myeloid leukemia: a subanalysis of the IRIS study. *Blood* 2008; 111(8): 4022-8.

[10] Singh, N., Kumar, L., et al. Drug monitoring of imatinib levels in patients undergoing therapy for chronic myeloid leukaemia: comparing plasma levels of responders and non-responders. *Eur. J. Clin. Pharmacol.* 2009; 65(6): 545-9.

[11] Sakai, M., Miyazaki, Y., et al. Long-term efficacy of imatinib in a practical setting is correlated with imatinib trough concentration that is influenced by body size: a report by the Nagasaki CML Study Group. *Int. J. Hematol.* 2009; 89(3): 319-25.

[12] Ishikawa, Y., Kiyoi, H., et al. Trough plasma concentration of imatinib reflects BCR-ABL kinase inhibitory activity and clinical response in chronic-phase chronic myeloid leukemia: a report from the BINGO study. *Cancer Sci.* 2010; 101(10): 2186-92.

[13] Awidi, A., Ayed, A. O., et al. Relationship of serum imatinib trough level and response in CML patients: long term follow-up. *Leuk. Res.* 2010; 34(12): 1573-5.

[14] Marin, D., Bazeos, A., et al. Adherence is the critical factor for achieving molecular responses in patients with chronic myeloid leukemia who achieve complete cytogenetic responses on imatinib. *J. Clin. Oncol.* 2010; 28(14): 2381-8.

[15] Takahashi, N., Wakita, H., et al. Correlation between imatinib pharmacokinetics and clinical response in Japanese patients with chronic-phase chronic myeloid leukemia. *Clin. Pharmacol. Ther.* 2010; 88(6): 809-13.

[16] Li-Wan-Po, A., Farndon, P., et al. Integrating pharmacogenetics and therapeutic drug monitoring: optimal dosing of imatinib as a case-example. *Eur. J. Clin. Pharmacol.* 2010; 66(4): 369-74.

[17] Sohn, S. K., Oh, S. J., et al. Trough plasma imatinib levels are correlated with optimal cytogenetic responses at 6 months after treatment with standard dose of imatinib in newly diagnosed chronic myeloid leukemia. *Leuk. Lymphoma* 2011; 52(6): 1024-9.

[18] Guilhot, F., Hughes, T. P., et al. Plasma exposure of imatinib and its correlation with clinical response in the Tyrosine Kinase Inhibitor Optimization and Selectivity Trial. *Haematologica* 2012; 97(5): 731-8.

[19] Koren-Michowitz, M., Volchek, Y., et al. Imatinib plasma trough levels in chronic myeloid leukaemia: results of a multicentre study CSTI571AIL11TGLIVEC. *Hematol. Oncol.* 2012.

[20] Zhong, J. S., Meng, F. Y., et al. Correlation between imatinib trough concentration and efficacy in Chinese chronic myelocytic leukemia patients. *Acta Haematol.* 2012; 127 (4): 221-7.

[21] Delbaldo, C., Chatelut, E., et al. Pharmacokinetic-pharmacodynamic relationships of imatinib and its main metabolite in patients with advanced gastrointestinal stromal tumors. *Clin. Cancer Res.* 2006; 12(20 Pt 1): 6073-8.

[22] Widmer, N., Decosterd, L. A., et al. Relationship of imatinib free plasma levels and target genotype with efficacy and tolerability. *Br. J. Cancer* 2008; 98(10): 1633-40.

[23] Demetri, G. D., Wang, Y., et al. Imatinib plasma levels are correlated with clinical benefit in patients with unresectable/metastatic gastrointestinal stromal tumors. *J. Clin. Oncol.* 2009; 27(19): 3141-7.

[24] Widmer, N. *Imatinib plasma concentrations variability in oncologic patients: Is imatinib a candidate drug for a therapeutic drug monitoring program?* Saarbrücken: LAP Lambert Academic Publishing; 2010.

[25] Klumpen, H. J., Samer, C. F., et al. Moving towards dose individualization of tyrosine kinase inhibitors. *Cancer Treat. Rev.* 2011; 37(4): 251-60.

[26] Peng, B., Dutreix, C., et al. Absolute bioavailability of imatinib (Glivec) orally versus intravenous infusion. *J. Clin. Pharmacol.* 2004; 44(2): 158-62.

[27] Peng, B., Lloyd, P., et al. Clinical pharmacokinetics of imatinib. *Clin. Pharmacokinet.* 2005; 44(9): 879-94.

[28] Gschwind, H. P., Pfaar, U., et al. Metabolism and disposition of imatinib mesylate in healthy volunteers. *Drug Metab. Dispos.* 2005; 33(10): 1503-12.

[29] Judson, I., Peiming, M., et al. Imatinib pharmacokinetics in patients with gastrointestinal stromal tumour: a retrospective population pharmacokinetic study over time. EORTC Soft Tissue and Bone Sarcoma Group. *Cancer Chemother. Pharmacol.* 2005; 55(4): 379-86.

[30] Schmidli, H., Peng, B., et al. Population pharmacokinetics of imatinib mesylate in patients with chronic-phase chronic myeloid leukaemia: results of a phase III study. *Br. J. Clin. Pharmacol.* 2005; 60(1): 35-44.

[31] Widmer, N., Decosterd, L. A., et al. Population Pharmacokinetics of imatinib and role of alpha-1-acid glycoprotein. *Br. J. Clin. Pharmacol.* 2006; 62(1): 97-112 [erratum: *Br. J. Clin. Pharmacol.* 2010; 70(2): 316].

[32] Petain, A., Kattygnarath, D., et al. Population pharmacokinetics and pharmacogenetics of imatinib in children and adults. *Clin. Cancer Res.* 2008; 14(21): 7102-9.

[33] Menon-Andersen, D., Mondick, J. T., et al. Population pharmacokinetics of imatinib mesylate and its metabolite in children and young adults. *Cancer Chemother. Pharmacol.* 2009; 63(2): 229-38.

[34] Yamakawa, Y., Hamada, A., et al. Association of genetic polymorphisms in the influx transporter SLCO1B3 and the efflux transporter ABCB1 with imatinib pharmacokinetics in patients with chronic myeloid leukemia. *Ther. Drug Monit.* 2011; 33(2): 244-50.

[35] Gotta, V., Buclin, T., et al. Systematic review of population pharmacokinetic analyses of imatinb and relationships with treatment outcome. *Ther. Drug Monit.* 2013; 35(2): 150-67.

[36] Cohen, M. H., Williams, G., et al. Approval summary for imatinib mesylate capsules in the treatment of chronic myelogenous leukemia. *Clin. Cancer Res.* 2002; 8(5): 935-42.

[37] Reckmann, A. H., Fischer, T., et al. Effect of food on STI571 Glivec pharmacokinetics and bioavailability. 37th Annual Meeting of the American Society of Clinical Oncology; San Francisco: *Proceedings - American Society of Clinical Oncology*; 2001; Abstr 1223.

[38] Singh, B. N., Malhotra, B. K. Effects of food on the clinical pharmacokinetics of anticancer agents: underlying mechanisms and implications for oral chemotherapy. *Clin. Pharmacokinet.* 2004; 43(15): 1127-56.

[39] Nikolova, Z., Peng, B., et al. Bioequivalence, safety, and tolerability of imatinib tablets compared with capsules. *Cancer Chemother. Pharmacol.* 2004; 53(5): 433-8.

[40] Sparano, B. A., Egorin, M. J., et al. Effect of antacid on imatinib absorption. *Cancer Chemother. Pharmacol.* 2009; 63(3): 525-8.

[41] Haouala, A., Widmer, N., et al. Prediction of free imatinib concentrations based on total plasma levels in GIST patients. *Br. J. Clin. Pharmacol.* 2013; 75(4): 1007-18.

[42] Yoo, C., Ryu, M. H., et al. Cross-sectional study of imatinib plasma trough levels in patients with advanced gastrointestinal stromal tumors: impact of gastrointestinal resection on exposure to imatinib. *J. Clin. Oncol.* 2010; 28(9): 1554-9.

[43] Gambacorti-Passerini, C., Zucchetti, M., et al. Alpha1 acid glycoprotein binds to imatinib (STI571) and substantially alters its pharmacokinetics in chronic myeloid leukemia patients. *Clin. Cancer Res.* 2003; 9(2): 625-32.

[44] Kretz, O., Weiss, H. M., et al. In vitro blood distribution and plasma protein binding of the tyrosine kinase inhibitor imatinib and its active metabolite, CGP74588, in rat, mouse, dog, monkey, healthy humans and patients with acute lymphatic leukaemia. *Br. J. Clin. Pharmacol.* 2004; 58(2): 212-6.

[45] Fitos, I., Visy, J., et al. Selective binding of imatinib to the genetic variants of human alpha1-acid glycoprotein. *Biochim. Biophys. Acta* 2006; 1760(11): 1704-12.

[46] Zsila, F., Fitos, I., et al. Determination of human serum alpha1-acid glycoprotein and albumin binding of various marketed and preclinical kinase inhibitors. *Curr. Med. Chem.* 2009; 16(16): 1964-77.

[47] Duche, J. C., Herve, F., et al. Study of the expression of the genetic variants of human alpha1-acid glycoprotein in healthy subjects using isoelectric focusing and immunoblotting. *J. Chromatogr. B Biomed. Sci. App.* 1998; 715(1): 103-9.

[48] Herve, F., Duche, J. C., et al. Changes in expression and microheterogeneity of the genetic variants of human alpha1-acid glycoprotein in malignant mesothelioma. *J. Chromatogr. B Biomed. Sci. App.* 1998; 715(1): 111-23.

[49] Mahon, F. X., Belloc, F., et al. MDR1 gene overexpression confers resistance to imatinib mesylate in leukemia cell line models. *Blood* 2003; 101(6): 2368-73.

[50] Widmer, N., Colombo, S., et al. Functional consequence of MDR1 expression on imatinib intracellular concentrations. *Blood* 2003; 102(3): 1142.

[51] Brendel, C., Scharenberg, C., et al. Imatinib mesylate and nilotinib (AMN107) exhibit high-affinity interaction with ABCG2 on primitive hematopoietic stem cells. *Leukemia* 2007; 21(6): 1267-75.

[52] Ozvegy-Laczka, C., Hegedus, T., et al. High-affinity interaction of tyrosine kinase inhibitors with the ABCG2 multidrug transporter. *Mol. Pharmacol.* 2004; 65(6): 1485-95.

[53] White, D. L., Saunders, V. A., et al. OCT-1-mediated influx is a key determinant of the intracellular uptake of imatinib but not nilotinib (AMN107): reduced OCT-1 activity is the cause of low in vitro sensitivity to imatinib. *Blood* 2006; 108(2): 697-704.

[54] Melo, J. V. Imatinib and ABCG2: who controls whom? *Blood* 2006; 108(4): 1116-7.

[55] Le Coutre, P., Kreuzer, K. A., et al. Pharmacokinetics and cellular uptake of imatinib and its main metabolite CGP74588. *Cancer Chemother. Pharmacol.* 2004; 53(4): 313-23.

[56] Breedveld, P., Pluim, D., et al. The effect of Bcrp1 (Abcg2) on the in vivo pharmacokinetics and brain penetration of imatinib mesylate (Gleevec): implications for the use of breast cancer resistance protein and P-glycoprotein inhibitors to enable the brain penetration of imatinib in patients. *Cancer Res.* 2005; 65(7): 2577-82.

[57] Bornhauser, M., Jenke, A., et al. CNS blast crisis of chronic myelogenous leukemia in a patient with a major cytogenetic response in bone marrow associated with low levels of imatinib mesylate and its N-desmethylated metabolite in cerebral spinal fluid. *Ann. Hematol.* 2004; 83(6): 401-2.

[58] Di Gion, P., Kanefendt, F., et al. Clinical pharmacokinetics of tyrosine kinase inhibitors: focus on pyrimidines, pyridines and pyrroles. *Clin. Pharmacokinet.* 2011; 50 (9): 551-603.

[59] Lyseng-Williamson, K., Jarvis, B. Imatinib. *Drugs* 2001; 61(12): 1765-74 [discussion 75-6].

[60] Morant, J., Ruppanner, H. *Compendium suisse des médicaments 2013.* Basel: Documed; 2012.

[61] Van Erp, N. P., Gelderblom, H., et al. Clinical pharmacokinetics of tyrosine kinase inhibitors. *Cancer Treat. Rev.* 2009; 35(8): 692-706.

[62] Rochat, B. Role of cytochrome P450 activity in the fate of anticancer agents and in drug resistance: focus on tamoxifen, paclitaxel and imatinib metabolism. *Clin. Pharmacokinet.* 2005; 44(4): 349-66.

[63] Rochat, B., Fayet, A., et al. Imatinib metabolite profiling in parallel to imatinib quantification in plasma of treated patients using liquid chromatography-mass spectrometry. *J. Mass Spectrom.* 2008; 43(6): 736-52.

[64] Levêque, D., Maloisel, F. Clinical pharmacokinetics of imatinib mesylate. *In Vivo* 2005; 19(1): 77-84.

[65] Rowland, M., Tozer, T. N. Distribution of drugs extensively bound to plasma protein. In: Rowland M, Tozer TN, editors. *Clinical pharmacokinetics: Concept and applications.* 4th ed. Baltimore: Lippincott, Wiliams and Wilkins; 2010. p. 695-702.

[66] Ramanathan, R. K., Egorin, M. J., et al. Phase I and pharmacokinetic study of imatinib mesylate in patients with advanced malignancies and varying degrees of liver dysfunction: a study by the National Cancer Institute Organ Dysfunction Working Group. *J. Clin. Oncol.* 2008; 26(4): 563-9.

[67] Judson, I. R. Imatinib for patients with liver or kidney dysfunction: no need to modify the dose. *J. Clin. Oncol.* 2008; 26(4): 521-2.

[68] Gibbons, J., Egorin, M. J., et al. Phase I and pharmacokinetic study of imatinib mesylate in patients with advanced malignancies and varying degrees of renal dysfunction: a study by the National Cancer Institute Organ Dysfunction Working Group. *J. Clin. Oncol.* 2008; 26(4): 570-6.

[69] Eechoute, K., Fransson, M. N., et al. A long-term prospective population pharmacokinetic study on imatinib plasma concentrations in GIST patients. *Clin. Cancer Res.* 2012; 18(20): 5780-7.

[70] Forrest, D. L., Trainor, S., et al. Cytogenetic and molecular responses to standard-dose imatinib in chronic myeloid leukemia are correlated with Sokal risk scores and duration of therapy but not trough imatinib plasma levels. *Leuk. Res.* 2009; 33(2): 271-5.
[71] Faber, E., Friedecky, D., et al. Imatinib trough plasma levels do not correlate with the response to therapy in patients with chronic myeloid leukemia in routine clinical setting. *Ann. Hematol.* 2012; 91(6): 923-9.
[72] Li, Q. B., Chen, C., et al. Imatinib plasma trough concentration and its correlation with characteristics and response in Chinese CML patients. *Acta Pharmacol. Sin.* 2010; 31 (8): 999-1004.
[73] Mahon, F. X., Molimard, M. Correlation between trough imatinib plasma concentration and clinical response in chronic myeloid leukemia. *Leuk. Res.* 2009; 33(8): 1147-8 [author reply 9-50].
[74] Branford, S., Rudzki, Z., et al. Detection of BCR-ABL mutations in patients with CML treated with imatinib is virtually always accompanied by clinical resistance, and mutations in the ATP phosphate-binding loop (P-loop) are associated with a poor prognosis. *Blood* 2003; 102(1): 276-83.
[75] Hughes, T., Deininger, M., et al. Monitoring CML patients responding to treatment with tyrosine kinase inhibitors: review and recommendations for harmonizing current methodology for detecting BCR-ABL transcripts and kinase domain mutations and for expressing results. *Blood* 2006; 108(1): 28-37.
[76] Debiec-Rychter, M., Sciot, R., et al. KIT mutations and dose selection for imatinib in patients with advanced gastrointestinal stromal tumours. *Eur. J. Cancer* 2006; 42(8): 1093-103.
[77] Cortes, J. E., Egorin, M. J., et al. Pharmacokinetic/pharmacodynamic correlation and blood-level testing in imatinib therapy for chronic myeloid leukemia. *Leukemia* 2009.
[78] Druker, B. J., Tamura, S., et al. Effects of a selective inhibitor of the Abl tyrosine kinase on the growth of Bcr-Abl positive cells. *Nat. Med.* 1996; 2(5): 561-6.
[79] Larson, R. A., Chia, Y. L., et al. Steady-state imatinib trough levels as well as dose interruptions are associated with clinical response (CCyR and MMR) and adverse events (AEs) in patients with chronic myeloid leukemia (CML) receiving IM as frontline therapy [abstract 2213]. *Blood* 2009; 114(22): 872.
[80] Blay, J. Y., Le Cesne, A., et al. Prospective multicentric randomized phase III study of imatinib in patients with advanced gastrointestinal stromal tumors comparing interruption versus continuation of treatment beyond 1 year: the French Sarcoma Group. *J. Clin. Oncol.* 2007; 25(9): 1107-13.
[81] Widmer, N., Decosterd, L. A., et al. Imatinib plasma levels: correlation with clinical benefit in GIST patients. *Br. J. Cancer* 2010; 102(7): 1198-9.
[82] Bui, B. N., Italiano, A., et al. Trough imatinib plasma levels in patients treated for advanced gastrointestinal stromal tumors evidence of large interpatient variations under treatment with standard doses. *J. Clin. Oncol.* 2008; 26(15S): 10564.
[83] Heinrich, M. C., Corless, C. L., et al. Molecular correlates of imatinib resistance in gastrointestinal stromal tumors. *J. Clin. Oncol.* 2006; 24(29): 4764-74.
[84] Heinrich, M. C., Owzar, K., et al. Correlation of kinase genotype and clinical outcome in the North American Intergroup Phase III Trial of imatinib mesylate for treatment of advanced gastrointestinal stromal tumor: CALGB 150105 Study by Cancer and

Leukemia Group B and Southwest Oncology Group. *J. Clin Oncol.* 2008; 26(33): 5360-7.

[85] Comparison of two doses of imatinib for the treatment of unresectable or metastatic gastrointestinal stromal tumors: a meta-analysis of 1,640 patients. *J. Clin. Oncol.* 2010; 28(7): 1247-53.

[86] Breccia, M., Cannella, L., et al. Cytogenetic and molecular responses in chronic phase chronic myeloid leukaemia patients receiving low dose of imatinib for intolerance to standard dose. *Hematol. Oncol.* 2010; 28(2): 89-92.

[87] Kobayashi, S., Kimura, F., et al. Efficacy of low-dose imatinib in chronic-phase chronic myelogenous leukemia patients. *Ann. Hematol.* 2009; 88(4): 311-5.

[88] Kimura, O., Yamamoto, O., et al. [Usefulness of low-dose and long-term administration of imatinib in patients with liver metastases of rectal GIST and GIST of stomach]. *Gan To Kagaku Ryoho* 2010; 37(12): 2285-7.

[89] Baccarani, M., Rosti, G., et al. Comparison of imatinib 400 mg and 800 mg daily in the front-line treatment of high-risk, Philadelphia-positive chronic myeloid leukemia: a European LeukemiaNet Study. *Blood* 2009; 113(19): 4497-504.

[90] Dasgupta, A. Clinical utility of free drug monitoring. *Clin. Chem. Lab. Med.* 2002; 40 (10): 986-93.

[91] Streit, F., Binder, L., et al. Use of total and unbound imatinib and metabolite LC-MS/MS assay to understand individual responses in CML and GIST patients. *Ther. Drug Monit.* 2011; 33(5): 632-43.

[92] Arellano, C., Gandia, P., et al. Determination of bound fraction of imatinib and N-desmethyl imatinib, Validation of an UPLC-MS/MS assay and ultrafiltration method. *J. Chromatogr. B Analyt. Technol. Biomed. Life Sci.* 2012; 907: 94-100.

[93] Haouala, A., Rumpold, H., et al. siRNA-mediated knock-down of P-glycoprotein expression reveals distinct cellular disposition of anticancer tyrosine kinases inhibitors. *Drug Metab. Lett.* 2010; 4(2): 114-9.

[94] Bouchet, S., Chauzit, E., et al. Simultaneous determination of nine tyrosine kinase inhibitors by 96-well solid-phase extraction and ultra performance LC/MS-MS. *Clin. Chim. Acta* 2011; 412(11-12): 1060-7.

[95] Decosterd, L. A., Dahmane, E., et al. Therapeutic drug monitoring of targeted anticancer therapy. Tyrosine kinase inhibitors and selective estrogen receptor modulators: A clinical pharmacology laboratory perspective. In: Xu, Q. A., Madden, T. L., editors. *LC-MS in Drug Bioanalysis*: Springer; 2012. p. 197-250.

[96] White, D. L., Saunders, V. A., et al. Most CML patients who have a suboptimal response to imatinib have low OCT-1 Activity. Higher doses of imatinib may overcome the negative impact of low OCT-1 Activity. *Blood* 2007.

[97] Widmer, N., Rumpold, H., et al. Resistance reversal by RNAi silencing of MDR1 in CML cells associated with increase in imatinib intracellular levels. *Leukemia* 2007; 21 (7): 1561-2 [author reply 2-4].

[98] White, D. L., Saunders, V. A., et al. OCT-1 activity measurement provides a superior imatinib response predictor than screening for single-nucleotide polymorphisms of OCT-1. *Leukemia* 2010; 24(11): 1962-5.

[99] White, D. L., Dang, P., et al. Functional activity of the OCT-1 protein is predictive of long-term outcome in patients with chronic-phase chronic myeloid leukemia treated with imatinib. *J. Clin. Oncol.* 2010; 28(16): 2761-7.

[100] Thomas, J., Wang, L., et al. Active transport of imatinib into and out of cells: implications for drug resistance. *Blood* 2004; 104(12): 3739-45.
[101] Crossman, L. C., Druker, B. J., et al. hOCT1 and resistance to imatinib. *Blood* 2005; 106(3): 1133-4 [author reply 4].
[102] Wang, L., Giannoudis, A., et al. Expression of the uptake drug transporter hOCT1 is an important clinical determinant of the response to imatinib in chronic myeloid leukemia. *Clin. Pharmacol. Ther.* 2008; 83(2): 258-64.
[103] Engler, J. R., Frede, A., et al. The poor response to imatinib observed in CML patients with low OCT-1 activity is not attributable to lower uptake of imatinib into their CD34+ cells. *Blood* 2010; 116(15): 2776-8.
[104] Rumpold, H., Wolf, A. M., et al. The role of P-glycoporotein in imatinib resistance. *Leukemia* 2006; 20(1): 144 [author reply 145].
[105] Shukla, S., Sauna, Z. E., et al. Evidence for the interaction of imatinib at the transport-substrate site(s) of the multidrug-resistance-linked ABC drug transporters ABCB1 (P-glycoprotein) and ABCG2. *Leukemia* 2008; 22(2): 445-7.
[106] Illmer, T., Schaich, M., et al. P-glycoprotein-mediated drug efflux is a resistance mechanism of chronic myelogenous leukemia cells to treatment with imatinib mesylate. *Leukemia* 2004; 18(3): 401-8.
[107] Rumpold, H., Wolf, A. M., et al. RNAi-mediated knockdown of P-glycoprotein using a transposon-based vector system durably restores imatinib sensitivity in imatinib-resistant CML cell lines. *Exp. Hematol.* 2005; 33(7): 767-75.
[108] Hirayama, C., Watanabe, H., et al. Constitutive overexpression of P-glycoprotein, rather than breast cancer resistance protein or organic cation transporter 1, contributes to acquisition of imatinib-resistance in K562 cells. *Pharm. Res.* 2008; 25(4): 827-35.
[109] Ferrao, P. T., Frost, M. J., et al. Overexpression of P-glycoprotein in K562 cells does not confer resistance to the growth inhibitory effects of imatinib (STI571) in vitro. *Blood* 2003; 102(13): 4499-503.
[110] Zong, Y., Zhou, S., et al. Loss of P-glycoprotein expression in hematopoietic stem cells does not improve responses to imatinib in a murine model of chronic myelogenous leukemia. *Leukemia* 2005; 19(9): 1590-6.
[111] Hatziieremia, S., Jordanides, N. E., et al. Inhibition of MDR1 does not sensitize primitive chronic myeloid leukemia CD34+ cells to imatinib. *Exp. Hematol.* 2009; 37 (6): 692-700.
[112] Lange, T., Gunther, C., et al. High levels of BAX, low levels of MRP-1, and high platelets are independent predictors of response to imatinib in myeloid blast crisis of CML. *Blood* 2003; 101(6): 2152-5.
[113] Dulucq, S., Bouchet, S., et al. Multidrug resistance gene (MDR1) polymorphisms are associated with major molecular responses to standard-dose imatinib in chronic myeloid leukemia. *Blood* 2008; 112(5): 2024-7.
[114] Burger, H., van Tol, H., et al. Imatinib mesylate (STI571) is a substrate for the breast cancer resistance protein (BCRP)/ABCG2 drug pump. *Blood* 2004; 104(9): 2940-2.
[115] Houghton, P. J., Germain, G. S., et al. Imatinib mesylate is a potent inhibitor of the ABCG2 (BCRP) transporter and reverses resistance to topotecan and SN-38 in vitro. *Cancer Res.* 2004; 64(7): 2333-7.

[116] Wolff, N. C., Randle, D. E., et al. Imatinib mesylate efficiently achieves therapeutic intratumor concentrations in vivo but has limited activity in a xenograft model of small cell lung cancer. *Clin. Cancer Res.* 2004; 10(10): 3528-34.

[117] Neef, M., Ledermann, M., et al. Oral imatinib treatment reduces early fibrogenesis but does not prevent progression in the long term. *J. Hepatol.* 2006; 44(1): 167-75.

[118] Haouala, A., Widmer, N., et al. Drug interactions with the tyrosine kinase inhibitors imatinib, dasatinib, and nilotinib. *Blood* 2011; 117(8): e75-87.

[119] Dutreix, C., Peng, B., et al. Pharmacokinetic interaction between ketoconazole and imatinib mesylate (Glivec) in healthy subjects. *Cancer Chemother. Pharmacol.* 2004; 54(4): 290-4.

[120] Cholongitas, E., Pipili, C., et al. Dermatitis after suspected imatinib-levothyroxine interaction in a patient with gastrointestinal stromal tumor. *Cancer Chemother. Pharmacol.* 2008; 61(6): 1083-4.

[121] De Groot, J. W., Zonnenberg, B. A., et al. Imatinib induces hypothyroidism in patients receiving levothyroxine. *Clin. Pharmacol. Ther.* 2005; 78(4): 433-8.

[122] Gambillara, E., Laffitte, E., et al. Severe pustular eruption associated with imatinib and voriconazole in a patient with chronic myeloid leukemia. *Dermatology* 2005; 211(4): 363-5.

[123] Zhou, S. F., Xue, C. C., et al. Clinically important drug interactions potentially involving mechanism-based inhibition of cytochrome P450 3A4 and the role of therapeutic drug monitoring. *Ther. Drug Monit.* 2007; 29(6): 687-710.

[124] Bilgi, N., Bell, K., et al. Imatinib and Panax ginseng: a potential interaction resulting in liver toxicity. *Ann. Pharmacother.* 2010; 44(5): 926-8.

[125] Van Erp, N. P., Gelderblom, H., et al. Influence of CYP3A4 inhibition on the steady-state pharmacokinetics of imatinib. *Clin. Cancer Res.* 2007; 13(24): 7394-400.

[126] Haouala, A., Widmer, N., et al. Cardiovascular drug interactions with tyrosine kinase inhibitors. *Cardiovasc. Med.* 2010; 13(5): 147-54.

[127] Azum, M., Nishioka, Y., et al. Role of alpha1-acid glycoprotein in therapeutic antifibrotic effects of imatinib with macrolides in mice. *Am. J. Respir. Crit. Care Med.* 2007; 176(12): 1243-50.

[128] Kajita, T., Higashi, Y., et al. Effect of imatinib mesilate on the disposition kinetics of ciclosporin in rats. *J. Pharm. Pharmacol.* 2006; 58(7): 997-1000.

[129] Yokota, A., Kimura, S., et al. INNO-406, a novel BCR-ABL/Lyn dual tyrosine kinase inhibitor, suppresses the growth of Ph+ leukemia cells in the central nervous system, and cyclosporine A augments its in vivo activity. *Blood* 2007; 109(1): 306-14.

[130] Tan, S. Y., Kan, E., et al. Metronidazole leads to enhanced uptake of imatinib in brain, liver and kidney without affecting its plasma pharmacokinetics in mice. *J. Pharm. Pharmacol.* 2011; 63(7): 918-25.

[131] Bolton, A. E., Peng, B., et al. Effect of rifampicin on the pharmacokinetics of imatinib mesylate (Gleevec, STI571) in healthy subjects. *Cancer Chemother. Pharmacol.* 2004; 53(2): 102-6.

[132] Pursche, S., Schleyer, E., et al. Influence of enzyme-inducing antiepileptic drugs on trough level of imatinib in glioblastoma patients. *Curr. Clin. Pharmacol.* 2008; 3(3): 198-203.

[133] Frye, R. F., Fitzgerald, S. M., et al. Effect of St John's wort on imatinib mesylate pharmacokinetics. *Clin. Pharmacol. Ther.* 2004; 76(4): 323-9.

[134] Smit, P. The influence of St. John's wort on the pharmacokinetics and protein binding of imatinib mesylate. *Pharmacotherapy* 2004; 24(11): 1508-14.
[135] O'Brien, S. G., Meinhardt, P., et al. Effects of imatinib mesylate (STI571, Glivec) on the pharmacokinetics of simvastatin, a cytochrome p450 3A4 substrate, in patients with chronic myeloid leukaemia. *Br. J. Cancer* 2003; 89(10): 1855-9.
[136] Wang, Y., Zhou, L., et al. Effects of imatinib (Glivec) on the pharmacokinetics of metoprolol, a CYP2D6 substrate, in Chinese patients with chronic myelogenous leukaemia. *Br. J. Clin. Pharmacol.* 2008; 65(6): 885-92.
[137] Demetri, G. D., Benjamin, R. S., et al. NCCN Task Force report: management of patients with gastrointestinal stromal tumor (GIST)--update of the NCCN clinical practice guidelines. *J. Natl. Compr. Canc. Netw.* 2007; 5(Suppl. 2): S1-29 [quiz S30].
[138] Kim, D. W., Tan, E. Y., et al. Effects of imatinib mesylate on the pharmacokinetics of paracetamol (acetaminophen) in Korean patients with chronic myelogenous leukaemia. *Br. J. Clin. Pharmacol.* 2011; 71(2): 199-206.
[139] Ridruejo, E., Cacchione, R., et al. Imatinib-induced fatal acute liver failure. *World J. Gastroenterol.* 2007; 13(48): 6608-111.
[140] Levine, A. M., Richardson, J. L., et al. Compliance with oral drug therapy in patients with hematologic malignancy. *J. Clin. Oncol.* 1987; 5(9): 1469-76.
[141] Feng, W., Henk, H., et al. Compliance and persistency with imatinib. *J. Clin. Oncol.* 2006; 24(18S): 6038.
[142] Tsang, J., Rudychev, I., et al. Prescription compliance and persistency in chronic myelogenous leukemia (CML) and gastrointestinal stromal tumor (GIST) patients (pts) on imatinib (IM). *J. Clin. Oncol.* 2006; 24 (18S): 6119.
[143] Wood, L. A review on adherence management in patients on oral cancer therapies. *Eur. J. Oncol. Nurs.* 2012; 16(4): 432-8.
[144] Noens, L., van Lierde, M. A., et al. Prevalence, determinants, and outcomes of nonadherence to imatinib therapy in patients with chronic myeloid leukemia: the ADAGIO study. *Blood* 2009; 113(22): 5401-11.
[145] Patrikidou, A., Chabaud, S., et al. Influence of imatinib interruption and rechallenge on the residual disease in patients with advanced GIST: results of the BFR14 prospective French Sarcoma Group randomised, phase III trial. *Ann. Oncol.* 2013; 24(4): 1087-93.
[146] Mahon, F. X., Rea, D., et al. Discontinuation of imatinib in patients with chronic myeloid leukaemia who have maintained complete molecular remission for at least 2 years: the prospective, multicentre Stop Imatinib (STIM) trial. *Lancet Oncol.* 2010; 11 (11): 1029-35.
[147] Goh, H. G., Kim, Y. J., et al. Previous best responses can be re-achieved by resumption after imatinib discontinuation in patients with chronic myeloid leukemia: implication for intermittent imatinib therapy. *Leuk. Lymphoma* 2009; 50(6): 944-51.
[148] Buclin, T., Gotta, V., et al. Monitoring drug therapy. *Br. J. Clin. Pharmacol.* 2012; 73 (6): 917-23.
[149] Glasziou, P., Irwig, L., et al. Monitoring in chronic disease: a rational approach. *BMJ* 2005; 330(7492): 644-8.
[150] Buclin, T., Widmer, N., et al. Who is in charge of assessing therapeutic drug monitoring? The case of imatinib. *Lancet Oncol.* 2011; 12(1): 9-11.

[151] Teng, J. F., Mabasa, V. H., et al. The role of therapeutic drug monitoring of imatinib in patients with chronic myeloid leukemia and metastatic or unresectable gastrointestinal stromal tumors. *Ther. Drug Monit.* 2012; 34(1): 85-97.

[152] Division of Clinical Pharmacology. University Hospital Center and University of Lausanne. I-COME: Imatinib COncentration Monitoring Evaluation: the clinical usefulness of "routine" versus "rescue" therapeutic drug monitoring (TDM) interventions in chronic myeloid leukaemia (CML) patients. ISRCTN; [updated August 18, 2009; cited 2012 October 10]; Available from: http://www.controlled-trials.com/ISRCTN31181395.

[153] Sarcoma Alliance for Research through Collaboration. Study of dose escalation versus no dose escalation of imatinib in metastatic gastrointestinal stromal tumors (GIST) patients. ClinicalTrials.gov; [updated July 20, 2011; cited 2012 October 10]; Available from: http://clinicaltrials.gov/ct2/show/NCT01031628.

[154] Mahon, F. X., Picard, S., et al. Use of therapeutic drug monitoring in CML patients on imatinib. *Blood* 2007; 110(5): 1701.

[155] Mahon, F. X. Pharmacologic monitoring and determinants of intracytoplasmic drug levels. *Best practice and research Clinical haematology* 2009; 22(3): 381-6.

[156] Gao, B., Yeap, S., et al. Evidence for therapeutic drug monitoring of targeted anticancer therapies. *J. Clin. Oncol.* 2012; 30(32): 4017-25.

[157] De Francia, S., D'Avolio, A., et al. New HPLC-MS method for the simultaneous quantification of the antileukemia drugs imatinib, dasatinib, and nilotinib in human plasma. *J. Chromatogr. B Analyt. Technol. Biomed. Life Sci.* 2009; 877(18-19): 1721-6.

[158] Haouala, A., Zanolari, B., et al. Therapeutic Drug Monitoring of the new targeted anticancer agents imatinib, nilotinib, dasatinib, sunitinib, sorafenib and lapatinib by LC tandem mass spectrometry. *J. Chromatogr. B Analyt. Technol. Biomed. Life Sci.* 2009; 877(22): 1982-96.

[159] Widmer, N., Béguin, A., et al. Determination of imatinib (Gleevec) in human plasma by solid-phase extraction-liquid chromatography-ultraviolet absorbance detection. *J. Chromatogr. B Analyt. Technol. Biomed. Life Sci.* 2004; 803(2): 285-92.

[160] Roth, O., Spreux-Varoquaux, O., et al. Imatinib assay by HPLC with photodiode-array UV detection in plasma from patients with chronic myeloid leukemia: Comparison with LC-MS/MS. *Clin. Chim. Acta* 2010; 411(3-4): 140-6.

[161] EUTOS for chronic myeloid leukemia shows improved management and dose optimization is required. *Future Oncol.* 2008; 4(6): 758.

[162] Wang, Y., Chia, Y. L., et al. A therapeutic drug monitoring algorithm for refining the imatinib trough level obtained at different sampling times. *Ther. Drug Monit.* 2009; 31 (5): 579-84.

[163] Gotta, V., Widmer, N., et al. Therapeutic drug monitoring of imatinib: bayesian and alternative methods to predict trough levels. *Clin. Pharmacokinet.* 2012; 51(3): 187-201.

[164] Judson, I. R. Therapeutic drug monitoring of imatinib - new data strengthen the case. *Clin. Cancer Res.* 2012; 18(20): 5517-9.

[165] D'Avoli, A., Simiele, M., et al. HPLC-MS method for the simultaneous quantification of the antileukemia drugs imatinib, dasatinib and nilotinib in human peripheral blood mononuclear cell (PBMC). *J. Pharm. Biomed. Anal.* 2012; 59: 109-16.

[166] Podsadecki, T. J., Vrijens, B. C., et al. "White coat compliance" limits the reliability of therapeutic drug monitoring in HIV-1-infected patients. *HIV Clin. Trials* 2008; 9(4): 238-46.

[167] Widmer, N., Gotta, V., et al. Tyrosine kinase inhibitors concentration monitoring in chronic myeloid leukemia. *Leuk. Res.* 2010; 34(6): 698-9.

In: Imatinib
Editors: Mojtaba Akhtari and Ihab Elhemaidi
ISBN: 978-1-62808-297-5

Chapter 3

Imatinib Mesylate: Clinical Application and Management

Shiksha Kedia, Manisha Pant, Pranab Sharma Acharya, Nilakantan Viswanathan, Meekoo Dhar and Vijaya Raj Bhatt*
Division of Hematology and Oncology, Department of Internal Medicine, University of Nebraska Medical Center, Nebraska Medical Center, Omaha, NE, US

History

The recognition that oncogenes code for protein tyrosine kinases (TK), and are potential cause of cancer was a turning point in the area of cancer research in 1980s. It was discovered that the TKs are involved in normal cellular signaling and their aberrancies can lead to cancers and other proliferative diseases. This understanding led to the series of experiments which resulted in the development of the tyrosine phosphorylation inhibitors (tryphostins), a low molecular weight antiproliferative agent specific for epidermal growth factor receptor. Later in 1990s, Brian Druker and Nicholas Lydon introduced imatinib as the first successful drug which targeted a specific oncogene product Bcr-Abl.

Chemical modification in its structure led to the enhanced cellular activity of imatinib against platelet derived growth factor receptor (PDGFR) TK and loss of serine/threonine kinase inhibition.

These modifications have also contributed to the inhibitory activity towards the cytoplasmic ABL TK and receptor KIT TK. Furthermore, the improved water solubility and oral bioavailability was the result of the addition of N-methylpiperazine ring. The discovery of imatinib in 1990s has revolutionized the treatment of chronic myeloid leukemia (CML) and other tumors and brought about a great surge of targeted therapies in the field of oncology [1, 2].

* Corresponding author: Vijaya Raj Bhatt. Division of Hematology and Oncology, Department of Internal Medicine, University of Nebraska Medical Center, 987680 Nebraska Medical Center, Omaha, NE, 68198-7680 US, E-mail: vijaya.bhatt@unmc.edu.

Chemical Structure

Formerly known as STI 571, imatinib mesylate is 4-[(4-methyl-1-piperazinyl) methyl]-N-[4-methyl-3-[[4-(3-pyridiny)-2-pyrimidynyl] amino] phenyl]benzamidemethanesulfonate with chemical formula of C29H31N7O.

The chemical structure is given below:

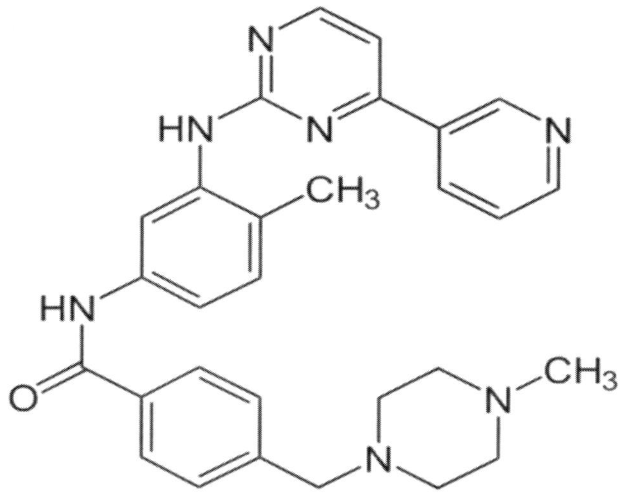

Source: Wikipedia, http://en.wikipedia.org/wiki/File:Imatinib.svg.

Imatinib Mesylate: Chemical Structure.

Mechanism of Action

TK is a constitutively active kinase that binds ATP (adenosine tri-phosphate) and transfers phosphate from ATP to tyrosine residues in various substrates. Such phosphorylation activates signal-transduction pathways that are vital for cellular growth, differentiation, and death [3]. TKs have a significant role in the pathogenesis of many tumors including CML, gastrointestinal stromal tumor (GIST), and dermatofibrosarcoma protuberans (DFSP). Imatinib is an inhibitor of several TKs such as Bcr-Abl, c-KIT and PDGFR-α and PDGFR-β. It competitively inhibits ATP binding, which leads to substrate phosphorylation and ultimately cellular proliferation [4-8].

Resistance

Based on the initial response to imatinib, resistance is divided as primary or secondary. Primary resistance is when a patient fails to achieve desired response when imatinib is used as initial modality for chronic phase CML. It occurs in up to 25 % of patients. It may be related to insufficient inhibition of the Bcr-Abl TK or decreased numbers of normal hematopoietic cells resulting in failure to recover normal blood counts [9].

Patients who have primary resistance and low trough levels of imatinib may benefit from dose increment [10]. Secondary resistance is defined as the relapse of disease after initial response to imatinib. It occurs in 80%, 50%, and 15% of patients with blast crisis, accelerated phase, and chronic phase of CML respectively at approximately two years [10-13]. Secondary resistance may be due to reactivation of Bcr-Abl signaling or activation of other signaling pathways such as Src kinase [9]. Bcr-Abl signaling may be reactivated due to Bcr-Abl overexpression, intra-cellular drug elimination via transmembrane transporters or more commonly, due to single nucleotide mutations in Bcr-Abl. Such mutations cause conformational changes to ATP- or imatinib-binding sites, activation loop or catalytic domain [14-18].

Although in-vitro Bcr-Abl activity assays, mutational screens and gene expression profiling are under investigation, no test can reliably predict the likelihood of resistance. If resistance is suspected, compliance to medication and possible drug interactions should be carefully reviewed. Serum drug level may guide further drug dosing [19]. Disease phase should be re-determined with repeat bone marrow biopsy and cytogenetic analysis. Mutational analysis of BCR-ABL gene and an early appraisal for possible allogeneic stem cell transplant should be considered.

Various strategies have been employed to overcome resistance including dose increment or a switch to another TKI or the use of non-TKI. CML patients, who have initially achieved a cytogenetic response and later lost it or in those without mutations unresponsive to imatinib, increasing the dose of imatinib to 600-800 mg daily can be helpful [20-22]. Nilotinib, with greater Bcr-Abl specificity and potency, has been approved for the treatment of imatinib–resistant or intolerant CML in chronic or accelerated phases [22]. Studies with Dasatinib [23. and Bosutinib [24, 25] in imatinib resistant cases have been promising. Omacetaxine, a non–TKI drug, has shown some response in imatinib-resistant cases as well as when multiple TKIs fail [26].

Dosing and Administration

Imatinib tablets should be administered orally with meal and a large glass of water, preferably at the same time every day. Doses below 600 mg are taken once daily. In children, it can be given once or twice daily. Imatinib tablets are coated with iron. Therefore, doses of 800 mg or above should be taken as 400 mg tablets rather than 100 mg tablets in order to reduce exposure to iron. If a dose is missed, the medication should be taken as soon as one remembers about it. If the time is close to the next dose, it is advisable to skip the missed dose and take the regular dose instead. Two doses should not be taken at the same time. The dose varies depending on the indication (table 1). Furthermore, the following conditions require dose modification.

Post Gastric Surgery

Imatinib absorption may be reduced after gastric surgery (bypass, major gastrectomy, or resection), therefore monitoring of trough concentration may be necessary [27].

Table 1. Imatinib indication and dosing [28]

Indication	Dose in Adult
CML* chronic phase	400 mg/day†
CML* in blast crisis, accelerated phase, or relapse after interferon-alpha therapy	600 mg/day
Relapsed or refractory philadelphia chromosome positive acute lymphoblastic leukemia	600 mg/day
Myelodysplastic/myeloproliferative diseases associated with PDGFR‡ gene re-arrangements	400 mg/day
Aggressive systemic mastocytosis without the D816V c-Kit mutation or with unknown mutational status	100 mg/day or 400 mg/day
Hypereosinophilic syndrome and/or chronic eosinophilic leukemia with FIP1L1-PDGFRα fusion kinase‡ and negative or unknown FIP1L1-PDGFRα fusion kinase‡	100 mg/day or 400 mg/day
Unresectable, recurrent and/or metastatic DFSP§	800 mg/day
c-KIT positive unresectable and/or metastatic malignant GIST‖	400 mg/day
Adjuvant therapy for c-KIT positive GIST‖	400 mg/day

*CML: chronic myeloid leukemia; †340 mg/m^2/day in children with chronic phase CML ‡PDGFR: platelet derived growth factor receptor; §DFSP: dermatofibrosarcoma protuberans; ‖GIST: gastrointestinal stromal tumor.

Hepatic Impairment

Mild to moderate hepatic impairment does not require dose adjustment, however, a reduction of total dose by 25 % is advisable in severe hepatic impairment [28]. Grade 3 and 4 imatinib-induced hepatotoxicity requires withholding medication until the toxicity is resolved (table 2). Then after, the medication may be resumed slowly depending on the initial severity of adverse events. Imatinib can safely be restarted in many patients; however recurrent hepatotoxicity may require permanent discontinuation of imatinib [29-32]. In few cases of recurrent hepatotoxicity, oral prednisone has been reported to allow safe resumption of imatinib [30, 33-36].

Renal Impairment

The dose of imatinib should be progressively reduced with the worsening degree of renal impairment (table 2). It should be used with extreme caution in patients with severe renal impairment, where doses above 100 mg is tolerated by only a limited number of patients [28].

Cytopenia

Myelosuppression from imatinib can be managed with temporary interruption in therapy (table 2).

Table 2. Dose Adjustment for Hepatotoxicity and Renal Toxicity [28]

Laboratory test	Initial recommended adjustments
Bilirubin >3x IULN* Or Transaminases>5 x IULN*	Withhold imatinib until Bilirubin decreases to <1.5 x IULN* and Transaminases <2.5 x IULN.* Imatinib may then be resumed at reduced daily dose. In children: resume at 260 mg/m²/day instead of 340mg/m²/day.
GFR † 40-59	Maximum dose 600 mg/day
GFR† 20-39	Decrease by 50 %
GFR† <20	Use with caution (<100mg/day)
ANC‡ <1.0 x 10^9/L and/or Platelets <50x 10^9/L	In general, stop Imatinib until ANC ≥ 1.5 x 10^9/L and platelets ≥ 75 x 10^9/L; then resume imatinib at previous or reduced dose§

*IULN: Institutional Upper Limit of Normal; †GFR: glomerular filtration rate; ‡ANC: Absolute neutrophil count; §cytopenia should not be related to underlying leukemia in case of CML in blast crisis or accelerated phase.

It can be restarted at the same dose if the absolute neutrophil count (ANC) recover to more than 1500/μL and platelet count recover to more than 100,000/μL within 4 weeks of interruption of the drug. With slower recovery of counts, imatinib should be started at a lower dose of 300mg/day and escalated if cell counts do not decline further. In accelerated phase and blast crisis of CML, interruption is only indicated in life threatening situation [28, 29].

Dose modification based on drug interactions: Imatinib is a competitive inhibitor of the multiple cytochrome P-450 isoenzymes. Various interactions are possible with a wide number of drugs and herbal products. This may result in resistance or toxicity and hence may require an adjustment in the prescribed dose [5].

Agents Inducing CYP3A Metabolism

Clearance of oral dose is increased by as much as 3.8 folds when imatinib is given with multiple doses of rifampin [37]. Other drugs such as carbamazepine, oxcarbamazepine, phenytoin, fosphenytoin, phenobarbital, primidone and St, john's Wort also lower the serum level of imatinib. Therefore, concomitant use of imatinib and enzyme inducing drugs should be avoided if possible. However, when these drugs have to be used simultaneously, imatinib dose should be increased by 50 % and clinical response should be carefully monitored. Doses of up to 600 mg twice daily have been given when strong CYP3A4 inducers are concomitantly used [28].

Agents Inhibiting CYP3A Metabolism

There is a significant increase in imatinib concentration when co-administered with enzyme inhibitors such as grape fruit juice, ketoconazole, itraconazole, clarithromycin, atazanavir, indinavir, nefazodone, nelfinavir, ritonavir, saquinavir, telithromycin, and voriconazole. This could potentially lead to imatinib toxicity [28]. Clinical signs of imatinib toxicity should be monitored in these patients.

Interactions with Drugs Metabolized by CYP3A4

Imatinib has been shown to inhibit CYP3A4 enzyme. Precautions should be taken when using imatinib with drugs having a narrow therapeutic index such as alfentanil, cyclosporine, diergotamine, ergotamine, fentanyl, pimozide, quinidine, sirolimus or tacrolimus.

Imatinib also enhances the plasma concentration of other drugs metabolized by CYP3A4 enzyme including benzodiazepines, dihydropyridine calcium channel blockers and few HMG-CoA reductase inhibitors (e.g. simvastatin) [28]. Clinical signs of toxicity of these specific drugs should be evaluated.

Warfarin is metabolized by CYP2C9 and CYP3A4. In patients that need anticoagulation, either standard heparin or low-molecular weight heparin should be used instead of warfarin if possible [28].

Interactions with Drugs Metabolized by CYP2D6

Imatinib has a weak inhibitory effect on drugs undergoing CYP2D6-mediated metabolism (e.g. metoprolol). Although dose adjustment is not necessary, caution is recommended [28].

Indications

There are several indications, for which imatinib has been approved by Food and Drug Administration. These are described below.

Newly Diagnosed Adult and Pediatric Patients with Philadelphia (Ph) Chromosome-Positive CML in the Chronic Phase: International Randomized Study of Interferon and STI571 trial among chronic phase CML patients showed a complete cytogenetic response (CCyR) rate at 18 months of 76% with imatinib (n=553) vs. 14% with interferon and cytarabine (n=553).

The rates of freedom from progression to the accelerated phase or blast phase were 97% vs 92% respectively [38]. After 5 years of follow up, the estimated cumulative rate of CCyR, progression-free survival (PFS) and overall survival (OS) was 87%, 83%, and 89% respectively with imatinib group (n=382) [4]. These studies have established imatinib as the standard of care for patients in chronic phase CML.

Advanced CML: A recent multicenter retrospective analysis (n=42) with accelerated phase CML showed an overall complete hematologic response (CHR) of 87.2% with 24-month OS and PFS of 87.8% and 87.2% respectively.

Though imatinib is a valuable option in CML-AP patients, the simultaneous presence of both additional chromosomal abnormalities and hematological acceleration at diagnosis is an unfavorable prognostic feature [39].

A prospective trial of imatinib (600 mg daily) in blast crisis CML (n=92) showed CHR of 26 %, CCyR of 10% and 18-month OS of 23% [40]. Thus, the role of imatinib in advanced stage CML, particularly blast crisis, is more of a "bridge" towards more definitive therapy such as allogeneic stem cell transplantation [41].

Adult Patients with Ph Chromosome–Positive Acute Lymphoblastic Leukemia: In CSTIBES02 (Concurrent intensive chemotherapy and imatinib before and after stem cell transplantation in newly diagnosed Philadelphia chromosome-positive acute lymphoblastic leukemia) trial (n=30), imatinib at doses of 400mg daily was used in a combination regimen in induction and consolidation therapy. The results from the trial showed a complete remission rate of 90 % as compared to 70% in ALL93 trial where same chemotherapy was used without imatinib [42].

Similar results with complete response rate of 90-95 % were seen in others studies [43-45]. Complete remission attained with imatinib is more durable when added to conventional chemotherapy regimen, thereby allowing more patients to proceed with post-remission therapy such as allogeneic hematopoietic cell transplantation. Furthermore, in elderly patients who are not a candidate for aggressive chemotherapy, combination therapy with imatinib and prednisone has been shown to result in a CHR rate of 100 % and an OS of 20 months (n=29) [46].

c-KIT-Positive Unresectable and/or Metastatic Malignant GIST: Imatinib (400 mg daily) has been shown to result in a PFS of 18 months and an OS of 55 months among patients with metastatic or surgically unresectable GIST. Escalation of dose to 400mg twice daily can be considered on progression of the disease [47].

Adjuvant Therapy for c-KIT-Positive GIST: A randomized multicenter trial showed 1-year recurrence free survival (RFS) of 98% with 1-year adjuvant imatinib therapy compared to 83% with placebo [48]. In another randomized multicenter study, adjuvant imatinib therapy for 36 months was shown to be better than imatinib for 12 months with a RFS of 65.6% versus 47.9% respectively [49].

Adult patients with myelodysplastic/myeloproliferative diseases (MDS/MPD) associated with PDGFR gene rearrangements: Imatinib has been shown to achieve a durable disease control with a median overall survival of 65 months in a study among MDS/MPD patients with PDGFR gene rearrangement [50].

Adult patients with aggressive systemic mastocytosis (ASM) without the D816V c-KIT mutation or unknown mutational status: Imatinib has been shown to be effective in ASM with imatinib-sensitive mutations and without D816V c-KIT mutation [51].

Adult patients with hypereosinophilic syndrome (HES) and/or chronic eosinophilic leukemia (CEL) who have FIP1L1-PDGFRα fusion kinase and for patients with HES and/or CEL who are FIP1L1-PDGFRα fusion kinase negative or unknown: Imatinib has been shown to induce a CHR in 14 days and complete molecular response in 9 months with an average duration of remission of 30 months [52]. The resistance to the drug is seen with a rare FIP1L1-PDGFRα point mutation causing loss of drug binding capacity [53].

Adult patients with unresectable, recurrent, and/or metastatic DFSP: In phase II B2225 trial, imatinib 400 mg twice daily resulted in a complete response rate of 33% and a partial response of 50% (n=12). The median time to disease progression was 24 months [54].

Isolated case reports with potential role of imatinib: Case series and isolated reports have been published showing potential role of imatinib in several other conditions such as recurrent and progressive meningioma, thymic carcinoma, cerebral langerhans cell histiocytosis, pulmonary arterial hypertension and diabetes mellitus [55-59]. These potential roles of imatinib require further substantiation.

Management of Adverse Effects

Common toxicities with imatinib are generally mild to moderate and tend to occur more frequently during the first 18 months of therapy. After the first 2 years or so, there is a decline in the frequency of new grade 3 and 4 adverse events [60].

In case of CML, adverse events requiring drug discontinuation is seen more commonly with blast crisis and accelerated phase compared with chronic phase [28].

Gastrointestinal Distress

Nausea and vomiting are among the most common side effects; in majority of the cases, they are mild and can be managed with antiemetics; however, they are also the most common dose limiting gastrointestinal side effects [29, 61] with 0.4-0.9 % cases being grade 3-4 [29]. Intake of imatinib with meals as well as splitting larger doses into bid regimens can reduce these side effects. Patients with history of hiatal hernia or esophagitis should take the medications two hours before bedtime. In severe cases antiemetics like prochlorperazine, or ondansetron can be used [62]. Diarrhea is also common and can be dose limiting. Local irritation as well as inhibition of the KIT of the Cajal cells of intestine may play a role in causing diarrhea. It is usually self-limiting and can be managed with antidiarrheal agents [29]. Gastrointestinal bleeding is more commonly associated with the treatment of GIST. It occurs in about 5% of cases with the risk being the highest in duodenal GIST and is often a result of tumor necrosis, bleeding from residual tumor or the development of gastric antral vascular ectasia [63].

Fluid Retention

Edema is reported in about 50 percent of cases [29] with 3-6% cases being more severe [64]. Although the majority of the cases are superficial such as periorbital edema or lower extremity edema, it can also cause ascites, pleural or pericardial effusion, pulmonary edema, cerebral edema and generalized anasarca [29]. The effects can be dose limiting and the severity is often dose-related [61]. The mechanism responsible for fluid retention is unknown. However, risk factors such as female sex, age >65, cardiac or renal insufficiency have been described [29]. Most of the cases of superficial edema are self-limiting and can be managed conservatively. Salt restriction can be helpful. Use of topical phenylephrine (0.25%) or hydrocortisone (1%) has shown to be beneficial in periorbital edema. However, severe cases not responding to diuretics may require discontinuation of the drug [29, 65]. With resolution of the symptoms, imatinib may be restarted at a lower dose with subsequent dose escalation along with the diuretics [29].

Hematological Toxicity

Imatinib suppresses normal hematopoiesis in only 10 to 20% of cases [66]. Significant myelosuppression is common in patients with CML especially with accelerated phase and blast crisis. In fact in CML, myelosuppression is a result of the therapeutic effect on the Ph-positive leukemic clone; blood counts eventually recover when imatinib is given as a continuous therapy [29]. In GIST, the incidence of myelosuppression primarily manifests as neutropenia [67]. Thrombocytopenia associated with the use of imatinib is proposed to be the result of the formation of anti-platelets antibodies [68].

Myelosupression is usually seen between 2 to 4 weeks in patients with blast crisis with later onset being common in accelerated and chronic phase [29].

Infectious complications are rarely (0.1 to 1%) seen despite neutropenia which is attributed to the lack of mucous membrane damage [29]. Herpes zoster infection is seen in about 2% of patients [69]. Intracranial and gastrointestinal hemorrhages can occur in patients in blast crisis with platelet counts less than 20,000. Imatinib-induced myelosuppression have been associated with mortality, which indicates that continued monitoring of peripheral blood counts is necessary [29].

Refer to 'cytopenia' under 'dosing and administration' section. The role of myeloid growth factors has not been well established in the treatment of myelosuppression [29].

Cardiotoxicity

Congestive heart failure as a result of imatinib is rare with an incidence of 0.04% per year [4] to 0.2% per year [70]. Inhibition of the ABL1 and KIT has been suggested as the potential cause of cardiotoxicity [71].

In patients with HES and cardiac involvement, cardiogenic shock and left ventricular dysfunction have been associated with the initiation of imatinib. The condition has been reported to be reversible with the administration of systemic steroids, circulatory support measures, and temporary withholding of imatinib [72].

This effect has also been observed with MDS/MPD and ASM associated with high eosinophil counts. A baseline Echocardiogram and troponin levels are obtained in these patients and any abnormalities require prophylactic treatment with steroids for one to two weeks along with imatinib therapy [28]. QT prolongation more than 500 ms is seen in 0.4% of cases, particularly among patients with preexisting cardiac conditions, thus requiring monitoring of such parameters among high-risk patients [73].

Hepatotoxicity

It can range from mild liver injury seen in about 10 % of cases to grade 3 and 4 hepatotoxicity which comprises of less than 5% of cases [4, 29, 74]. The toxicity usually manifests in early months of therapy but can be seen up to 22 weeks or even longer [29, 33, 75]. Although not very clear, drug-induced hypersensitivity have been postulated as the mechanism of the injury [29, 75].

Most cases are benign requiring no dose adjustment, but severe cases of hepatotoxicity can necessitate dose reduction or discontinuation of the drug [74]. After the discontinuation of imatinib, liver function tests often normalize in about 7 weeks but recovery can also take up to 20 weeks [74]. Avoiding the use of alcohol and acetaminophen hastens recovery [29, 33, 75]. With persistence of grade 2 toxicity despite adequate measures, further evaluation with screening for viral hepatitis, ferritin levels, alpha 1 antitrypsin level, or a liver biopsy may be indicated [29]. Also refer to 'hepatic impairment' under 'dosing and administration' section.

Renal Toxicity and Electrolyte Abnormalities

The decline in glomerular filtration rate and the development of chronic renal failure can be seen in up to 12 % of patients on imatinib [76]. This may be the result of PDGFR inhibition or altered processing of calcium and phosphorus [77].

Also refer to 'renal impairment' under 'dosing and administration' section. Hypophosphatemia [78] and hypocalcemia [79] can also be seen in a small number of patients on imatinib. Hypokalemia is seen in 13 % of cases but its causal relationship with imatinib has not been established [28].

Musculoskeletal Effects

Approximately one-third of the patients complain of fatigue and muscle cramps involving the calves, thighs, hands and feet. The use of calcium and magnesium supplementation as well as quinine may alleviate muscle cramps.

Arthralgia and bone pain mostly affecting tibia, femur, hip and knee are seen in 20 to 30% of patients, particularly during the first month of therapy.

These side effects often resolve within few months and oral analgesics (such as NSAIDS or opioids) can be helpful [29]. Imatinib can also result in the inhibition of bone remodeling [78] as well as an increase in the creatine kinase level and rhabdomyolysis [28, 80] in a small number of patients.

Dermatological Effects

Drug-induced rash occurs in about 30 % patients and can be dose limiting [81]. It manifests as pruritic, erythematous, maculopapular rash, mostly on the arms and the trunk and less frequently on the face [29]. Urticarial eruptions in patients with high basophil counts, alopecia, hyperpigmentation and repigmentation of hair [82], generalized exanthematous pustulosis [83], desquamating lesions including Steven Johnson Syndrome [84] have also been reported.

However, the majority of the cases is mild and benefit from the use of antihistamines or topical steroid. Severe cases may require systemic steroids and interruption of imatinib [29]. Prophylactic use of antihistamine is beneficial in some patients with high basophil counts (>20%) [29].

Effects on Endocrine System

Alteration in thyroid function has been seen in 25 % of cases treated with imatinib, however, most of the cases are subclinical and transient [85]. Hypothyroidism has been reported in thyroidectomy patients undergoing levothyroxine replacement during treatment with imatinib [86]. Gynecomastia (2-18% of cases) [87], cases of oligospermia [88] and primary ovarian insufficiency [89] are also reported.

Weight Gain

Twelve percent of the patients had weight gain in phase 3 trials, which was attributed partly to fluid retention and partly to the discontinuation of interferon with a return of normal appetite [29].

Development of Secondary Tumors

Several cases of secondary malignancies have been reported in association with the use of imatinib [90], however, the casual relationship have not been established. In fact a large study failed to show an increased risk of cancer in association with the use of imatinib [91].

Adverse Effects in Pediatric Age Group

Overall, imatinib is well tolerated with a relatively low incidence of grade 3 and 4 toxicity [92]. Of special concern in this age group is the risk of growth deceleration. Although the mechanism is not very clear, it is suggested that imatinib affects the production of insulin-like growth factor-1and inhibits a tyrosine kinase receptor known to regulate chondrocyte proliferation and activity [93, 94].

Safety during Pregnancy and Lactation

Imatinib is classified as a category D drug with positive evidence of fetal risk in both animal and human studies. Spontaneous abortion, gut mal-rotations and congential abnormalities including skeletal malformation, hypospadias, hypoplastic lung, and structural CNS abnormalities have been reported. Limited trials and anecdotal reports have not shown reduced sperm count or infertility in men. However, few reports of abortions, intrauterine death and gut malrotation have been published with the paternal use of imatinib [95-97]. Hence, highly effective contraception is recommended for all women and the female partners of men taking imatinib.

Imatinib and its active metabolite can enter breast milk. Up to 10% of therapeutic maternal dose could potentially be received by breast-fed infants. Withholding breast feeding or avoiding treatment during periods of breast feeding should be based on expected therapeutic benefits to the mother [28].

Other Adverse Effects

Many other side effects such as pyrexia, rigors, night sweats, weakness, pruritus, insomnia, depression, anxiety, headache, dizziness, dry mouth, anorexia, dyspepsia, sore throat, upper respiratory tract infection, nasopharyngitis, cough and dyspnea are reported but their causal relationship with imatinib have not been established [29].

Monitoring with Imatinib

In addition to regular clinical evaluation, therapy with imatinib require following parameters to be monitored.

Weight: Patients should be weighed regularly for signs and symptoms of fluid retention. An unexpected rapid weight gain requires careful assessment [28].

Complete blood count (CBC): It should be monitored weekly in patients with chronic-phase CML during the first month of imatinib therapy. In the absence of significant myelosuppression (ANC ≤1,500/µL or platelet count ≤100,000/µL), CBC can be monitored every 2 weeks until 12 weeks of therapy. Thereafter, it can be monitored monthly or even less frequently, depending on the stability of the counts and the disease. For patients in accelerated phase or blast crisis of CML, CBCs should be monitored more closely with initial monitoring done at least weekly [29].

Liver Function Test (LFT): It is recommended to perform a baseline LFTs before treatment and monthly LFTs thereafter [28].

Calcium, phosphorous, parathyroid hormone and Vitamin D levels: These tests may be done every 4 weeks during early periods of imatinib therapy. With sustained disturbances in these levels, bone densitometry may be indicated [73].

Thyroid function test: Regular monitoring is important especially for patients who are on levothyroxine treatment [85].

Creatinine Kinase: Monitoring should be considered in patients with muscle cramps [80].

Left Ventricular Ejection fraction and EKG- This is particularly important in patients with pre-existing cardiac conditions [73].

References

[1] Levitzki, A. Tyrosine kinases as targets for cancer therapy. *Eur. J. Cancer.* [Review]. 2002 Sep.;38 Suppl. 5:S11-8.

[2] Yaish, P., Gazit, A., Gilon, C., Levitzki, A. Blocking of EGF-dependent cell proliferation by EGF receptor kinase inhibitors. *Science.* [Comparative Study]. 1988 Nov. 11;242(4880):933-5.

[3] Kolibaba, K. S., Druker, B. J. Protein tyrosine kinases and cancer. *Biochim. Biophys. Acta.* [Review]. 1997 Dec. 9;1333(3):F217-48.

[4] Druker, B. J., Guilhot, F., O'Brien, S. G., Gathmann, I., Kantarjian, H., Gattermann, N., et al. Five-year follow-up of patients receiving imatinib for chronic myeloid leukemia. *N Engl. J. Med.* 2006 Dec. 7;355(23):2408-17.

[5] Peng, B., Lloyd, P., Schran, H. Clinical pharmacokinetics of imatinib. *Clin. Pharmacokinet.* 2005;44(9):879-94.

[6] Deininger, M., Buchdunger, E., Druker, B. J. The development of imatinib as a therapeutic agent for chronic myeloid leukemia. *Blood.* 2005 Apr. 1;105(7):2640-53.

[7] Capdeville, R., Buchdunger, E., Zimmermann, J., Matter, A. Glivec (STI571, imatinib), a rationally developed, targeted anticancer drug. *Nat. Rev. Drug Discov.* 2002 Jul.;1(7): 493-502.

[8] Mauro, M. J., Druker, B. J. STI571: targeting BCR-ABL as therapy for CML. *Oncologist*. [Review]. 2001;6(3):233-8.

[9] Milojkovic, D., Apperley, J. Mechanisms of Resistance to Imatinib and Second-Generation Tyrosine Inhibitors in Chronic Myeloid Leukemia. *Clin. Cancer Res*. 2009 Dec. 15;15(24):7519-27.

[10] Kantarjian, H. M., Talpaz, M., O'Brien, S., Giles, F., Garcia-Manero, G., Faderl, S., et al. Dose escalation of imatinib mesylate can overcome resistance to standard-dose therapy in patients with chronic myelogenous leukemia. *Blood*. 2003 Jan. 15;101 (2): 473-5.

[11] O'Dwyer, M. E., Mauro, M. J., Blasdel, C., Farnsworth, M., Kurilik, G., Hsieh, Y. C., et al. Clonal evolution and lack of cytogenetic response are adverse prognostic factors for hematologic relapse of chronic phase CML patients treated with imatinib mesylate. *Blood*. 2004 Jan. 15;103(2):451-5.

[12] Kantarjian, H., Talpaz, M., O'Brien, S., Giles, F., Rios, M. B., White, K., et al. Prediction of initial cytogenetic response for subsequent major and complete cytogenetic response to imatinib mesylate therapy in patients with Philadelphia chromosome-positive chronic myelogenous leukemia. *Cancer*. 2003 May 1;97(9):2225-8.

[13] Soverini, S., Martinelli, G., Rosti, G., Bassi, S., Amabile, M., Poerio, A., et al. ABL mutations in late chronic phase chronic myeloid leukemia patients with up-front cytogenetic resistance to imatinib are associated with a greater likelihood of progression to blast crisis and shorter survival: a study by the GIMEMA Working Party on Chronic Myeloid Leukemia. *J. Clin. Oncol*. 2005 Jun. 20;23(18):4100-9.

[14] Kantarjian, H. M., Talpaz, M., Giles, F., O'Brien, S., Cortes, J. New insights into the pathophysiology of chronic myeloid leukemia and imatinib resistance. *Ann. Intern. Med*. 2006 Dec. 19;145(12):913-23.

[15] White, D. L., Dang, P., Engler, J., Frede, A., Zrim, S., Osborn, M., et al. Functional activity of the OCT-1 protein is predictive of long-term outcome in patients with chronic-phase chronic myeloid leukemia treated with imatinib. *J. Clin. Oncol*. 2010 Jun. 1;28(16):2761-7.

[16] Jabbour, E., Cortes, J. E., Giles, F. J., O'Brien, S., Kantarjian, H. M. Current and emerging treatment options in chronic myeloid leukemia. *Cancer*. [Research Support, Non-US Gov't Review]. 2007 Jun. 1;109(11):2171-81.

[17] Gorre, M. E., Mohammed, M., Ellwood, K., Hsu, N., Paquette, R., Rao, P. N., et al. Clinical resistance to STI-571 cancer therapy caused by BCR-ABL gene mutation or amplification. *Science*. [Comment Research Support, Non-US Gov't Research Support, US Gov't, P.H.S.]. 2001 Aug. 3;293(5531):876-80.

[18] O'Hare, T., Eide, C. A., Deininger, M. W. Bcr-Abl kinase domain mutations, drug resistance, and the road to a cure for chronic myeloid leukemia. *Blood*. 2007 Oct. 1;110 (7):2242-9.

[19] Awidi, A., Salem, I. I., Najib, N., Mefleh, R., Tarawneh, B. Determination of imatinib plasma levels in patients with chronic myeloid leukemia by high performance liquid chromatography-ultraviolet detection and liquid chromatography-tandem mass spectrometry: methods' comparison. *Leuk. Res*. 2010 Jun.;34(6):714-7.

[20] Kantarjian, H. M., Larson, R. A., Guilhot, F., O'Brien, S. G., Mone, M., Rudoltz, M., et al. Efficacy of imatinib dose escalation in patients with chronic myeloid leukemia in chronic phase. *Cancer*. 2009 Feb. 1;115(3):551-60.

[21] Jabbour, E., Kantarjian, H. M., Jones, D., Shan, J., O'Brien, S., Reddy, N., et al. Imatinib mesylate dose escalation is associated with durable responses in patients with chronic myeloid leukemia after cytogenetic failure on standard-dose imatinib therapy. *Blood*. 2009 Mar. 5;113(10):2154-60.

[22] Jabbour, E., Parikh, S. A., Kantarjian, H., Cortes, J. Chronic myeloid leukemia: mechanisms of resistance and treatment. *Hematol. Oncol. Clin. North Am*. 2011 Oct.;25 (5):981-95, v.

[23] Cortes, J. E., Jones, D., O'Brien, S., Jabbour, E., Ravandi, F., Koller, C., et al. Results of dasatinib therapy in patients with early chronic-phase chronic myeloid leukemia. *J. Clin. Oncol*. 2010 Jan. 20;28(3):398-404.

[24] Cortes, J., Kantarjian, H. M., Kim, D.-W., Khoury, H. J., Turkina, A. G., Shen, Z.-X., et al. Efficacy and Safety of Bosutinib (SKI-606) in Patients with Chronic Phase (CP) Ph+ Chronic Myelogenous Leukemia (CML) with Resistance or Intolerance to Imatinib. *ASH Annual Meeting Abstracts*. 2008 December 5, 2008;112(11):1098.

[25] Gambacorti-Passerini, C., Kantarjian, H., Bruemmendorf, T., Martinelli, G., Baccarani, M., Fischer, T., et al. Bosutinib (SKI-606) Demonstrates Clinical Activity and Is Well Tolerated among Patients with AP and BP CML and Ph+ ALL. *ASH Annual Meeting Abstracts*. 2007 December 12, 2007;110(11):473.

[26] Cortes-Franco, J., Raghunadharao, D., Parikh, P., Wetzler, M., Lipton, J. H., Jones, D., et al. Safety and Efficacy of Subcutaneous-Administered Omacetaxine Mepesuccinate in Chronic Myeloid Leukemia (CML) Patients Who Are Resistant or Intolerant to Two or More Tyrosine Kinase Inhibitors - Results of A Multicenter Phase 2/3 Study. *ASH Annual Meeting Abstracts*. 2009 December 11, 2009;114(22):861.

[27] Lium, H., Artz, A. S. Reduction of imatinib absorption after gastric bypass surgery. *Leuk. Lymphoma*. 2011 Feb;52(2):310-3.

[28] Gleevec [Package Insert]. Pamphlet. East Hanover, New Jersey 07936: Novartis Pharmaceuticals Corporation; 2012.

[29] Deininger, M. W., O'Brien, S. G., Ford, J. M., Druker, B. J. Practical management of patients with chronic myeloid leukemia receiving imatinib. *J. Clin. Oncol*. 2003 Apr. 15;21(8):1637-47.

[30] Ferrero, D., Pogliani, E. M., Rege-Cambrin, G., Fava, C., Mattioli, G., Dellacasa, C., et al. Corticosteroids can reverse severe imatinib-induced hepatotoxicity. *Haematologica*. 2006 Jun.;91(6 Suppl.):ECR27.

[31] James, C., Trouette, H., Marit, G., Cony-Makhoul, P., Mahon, F. X. Histological features of acute hepatitis after imatinib mesylate treatment. *Leukemia*. 2003 May;17 (5):978-9.

[32] Rocca, P., El Jastimi, S., Troncy, J., Scoazec, J. Y., Boucher, A., Vial, T., et al. [Imatinib mesylate-induced acute cytolytic hepatitis]. *Gastroenterol. Clin. Biol*. 2004 Oct.;28(10 Pt 1):918-9.

[33] Asnacios, A., Naveau, S., Perlemuter, G. Gastrointestinal toxicities of novel agents in cancer therapy. *Eur. J. Cancer*. 2009 Sep.;45 Suppl. 1:332-42.

[34] Gupta, S., Bhatt, V. R., Varma, S. Recurrent imatinib-induced hepatotoxicity in a chronic myeloid leukaemia patient successfully managed with prednisone. *BMJ Case Rep*. 2011;2011.

[35] Yamazaki, R., Okamoto, S., Chen, C. K., Tada, S., Saito, H., Shibata, R., et al. Successful management of liver injury caused by imatinib mesylate in a patient with previously untreated chronic myelogenous leukemia in the chronic phase. *Leuk. Lymphoma*. 2006 Jul.;47(7):1427-30.

[36] Ikuta, K., Torimoto, Y., Jimbo, J., Inamura, J., Shindo, M., Sato, K., et al. Severe hepatic injury caused by imatinib mesylate administered for the treatment of chronic myeloid leukemia and the efficacy of prednisolone for its management. *Int. J. Hematol*. 2005 Nov.;82(4):343-6.

[37] Bolton, A. E., Peng, B., Hubert, M., Krebs-Brown, A., Capdeville, R., Keller, U., et al. Effect of rifampicin on the pharmacokinetics of imatinib mesylate (Gleevec, STI571) in healthy subjects. *Cancer Chemother. Pharmacol*. 2004 Feb.;53(2):102-6.

[38] O'Brien, S. G., Guilhot, F., Larson, R. A., Gathmann, I., Baccarani, M., Cervantes, F., et al. Imatinib compared with interferon and low-dose cytarabine for newly diagnosed chronic-phase chronic myeloid leukemia. *N Engl. J. Med*. 2003 Mar. 13;348(11):994-1004.

[39] Rea, D., Etienne, G., Nicolini, F., Cony-Makhoul, P., Johnson-Ansah, H., Legros, L., et al. First-line imatinib mesylate in patients with newly-diagnosed accelerated phase-chronic myeloid leukemia. *Leukemia*. 2012 Mar. 30.

[40] Palandri, F., Castagnetti, F., Testoni, N., Luatti, S., Marzocchi, G., Bassi, S., et al. Chronic myeloid leukemia in blast crisis treated with imatinib 600 mg: outcome of the patients alive after a 6-year follow-up. *Haematologica*. 2008 Dec.;93(12):1792-6.

[41] Schiffer, C. A. BCR-ABL tyrosine kinase inhibitors for chronic myelogenous leukemia. *N Engl. J. Med*. [Review]. 2007 Jul. 19;357(3):258-65.

[42] Ribera, J. M., Oriol, A., Gonzalez, M., Vidriales, B., Brunet, S., Esteve, J., et al. Concurrent intensive chemotherapy and imatinib before and after stem cell transplantation in newly diagnosed Philadelphia chromosome-positive acute lymphoblastic leukemia. Final results of the CSTIBES02 trial. *Haematologica*. 2010 Jan.;95(1):87-95.

[43] Yanada, M., Takeuchi, J., Sugiura, I., Akiyama, H., Usui, N., Yagasaki, F., et al. High complete remission rate and promising outcome by combination of imatinib and chemotherapy for newly diagnosed BCR-ABL-positive acute lymphoblastic leukemia: a phase II study by the Japan Adult Leukemia Study Group. *J. Clin. Oncol*. 2006 Jan. 20; 24(3):460-6.

[44] Thomas, D. A., Faderl, S., Cortes, J., O'Brien, S., Giles, F. J., Kornblau, S. M., et al. Treatment of Philadelphia chromosome-positive acute lymphocytic leukemia with hyper-CVAD and imatinib mesylate. *Blood*. 2004 Jun. 15;103(12):4396-407.

[45] Wassmann, B., Pfeifer, H., Goekbuget, N., Beelen, D. W., Beck, J., Stelljes, M., et al. Alternating versus concurrent schedules of imatinib and chemotherapy as front-line therapy for Philadelphia-positive acute lymphoblastic leukemia (Ph+ ALL). *Blood*. 2006 Sep. 1;108(5):1469-77.

[46] Vignetti, M., Fazi, P., Cimino, G., Martinelli, G., Di Raimondo, F., Ferrara, F., et al. Imatinib plus steroids induces complete remissions and prolonged survival in elderly Philadelphia chromosome-positive patients with acute lymphoblastic leukemia without

additional chemotherapy: results of the Gruppo Italiano Malattie Ematologiche dell'Adulto (GIMEMA) LAL0201-B protocol. *Blood.* 2007 May 1;109(9):3676-8.

[47] Blanke, C. D., Rankin, C., Demetri, G. D., Ryan, C. W., von Mehren, M., Benjamin, R. S., et al. Phase III randomized, intergroup trial assessing imatinib mesylate at two dose levels in patients with unresectable or metastatic gastrointestinal stromal tumors expressing the kit receptor tyrosine kinase: S0033. *J. Clin. Oncol.* 2008 Feb. 1;26(4): 626-32.

[48] Dematteo, R. P., Ballman, K. V., Antonescu, C. R., Maki, R. G., Pisters, P. W., Demetri, G. D., et al. Adjuvant imatinib mesylate after resection of localised, primary gastrointestinal stromal tumour: a randomised, double-blind, placebo-controlled trial. *Lancet.* 2009 Mar. 28;373(9669):1097-104.

[49] Joensuu, H., Eriksson, M., Sundby Hall, K., Hartmann, J. T., Pink, D., Schutte, J., et al. One vs three years of adjuvant imatinib for operable gastrointestinal stromal tumor: a randomized trial. *JAMA.* 2012 Mar. 28;307(12):1265-72.

[50] David, M., Cross, N. C., Burgstaller, S., Chase, A., Curtis, C., Dang, R., et al. Durable responses to imatinib in patients with PDGFRB fusion gene-positive and BCR-ABL-negative chronic myeloproliferative disorders. *Blood.* 2007 Jan. 1;109(1):61-4.

[51] Pardanani, A. Systemic mastocytosis in adults: 2012 Update on diagnosis, risk stratification, and management. *Am. J. Hematol.* [Review]. 2012 Apr.;87(4):401-11.

[52] Helbig, G., Moskwa, A., Hus, M., Piszcz, J., Swiderska, A., Urbanowicz, A., et al. Clinical characteristics of patients with chronic eosinophilic leukaemia (CEL) harbouring FIP1L1-PDGFRA fusion transcript--results of Polish multicentre study. *Hematol. Oncol.* [Multicenter Study Research Support, Non-U S Gov't]. 2010;28(2):93-7.

[53] Valent, P. Pathogenesis, classification, and therapy of eosinophilia and eosinophil disorders. *Blood reviews.* [Review]. 2009 Jul.;23(4):157-65.

[54] Heinrich, M. C., Joensuu, H., Demetri, G. D., Corless, C. L., Apperley, J., Fletcher, J. A., et al. Phase II, open-label study evaluating the activity of imatinib in treating life-threatening malignancies known to be associated with imatinib-sensitive tyrosine kinases. *Clin. Cancer Res.* 2008 May 1;14(9):2717-25.

[55] Reardon, D. A., Norden, A. D., Desjardins, A., Vredenburgh, J. J., Herndon, J. E., 2nd, Coan, A., et al. Phase II study of Gleevec(R) plus hydroxyurea (HU) in adults with progressive or recurrent meningioma. *J. Neurooncol.* [Clinical Trial, Phase II Multicenter Study Research Support, N.I.H., Extramural Research Support, Non-US Gov't]. 2012 Jan.;106(2):409-15.

[56] Strobel, P., Hartmann, M., Jakob, A., Mikesch, K., Brink, I., Dirnhofer, S., et al. Thymic carcinoma with overexpression of mutated KIT and the response to imatinib. *N Engl. J. Med.* [Case Reports Letter]. 2004 Jun. 17;350(25):2625-6.

[57] Montella, L., Insabato, L., Palmieri, G. Imatinib mesylate for cerebral Langerhans'-cell histiocytosis. *N Engl. J. Med.* [Case Reports Letter]. 2004 Sep. 2;351(10):1034-5.

[58] Ghofrani, H. A., Seeger, W., Grimminger, F. Imatinib for the treatment of pulmonary arterial hypertension. *N Engl. J. Med.* 2005 Sep. 29;353(13):1412-3.

[59] Veneri, D., Franchini, M., Bonora, E. Imatinib and regression of type 2 diabetes. *N Engl. J. Med.* [Case Reports Letter]. 2005 Mar. 10;352(10):1049-50.

[60] Moen, M. D., McKeage, K., Plosker, G. L., Siddiqui, M. A. Imatinib: a review of its use in chronic myeloid leukaemia. *Drugs.* 2007;67(2):299-320.

[61] Sawyers, C. L., Hochhaus, A., Feldman, E., Goldman, J. M., Miller, C. B., Ottmann, O. G., et al. Imatinib induces hematologic and cytogenetic responses in patients with chronic myelogenous leukemia in myeloid blast crisis: results of a phase II study. *Blood.* 2002 May 15;99(10):3530-9.
[62] Guilhot, F. Indications for imatinib mesylate therapy and clinical management. *Oncologist.* 2004;9(3):271-81.
[63] Saad Aldin, E., Mourad, F., Tfayli, A. Gastric Antral Vascular Ectasia in a Patient with GIST after Treatment with Imatinib: Case Report and Literature Review. *Jpn. J. Clin. Oncol.* 2012 Mar. 15.
[64] Savage, D. G., Antman, K. H. Imatinib mesylate--a new oral targeted therapy. *N Engl. J. Med.* 2002 Feb. 28;346(9):683-93.
[65] Cervantes, F., Mauro, M. Practical management of patients with chronic myeloid leukemia. *Cancer.* 2011 Oct. 1;117(19):4343-54.
[66] Druker, B. J., Tamura, S., Buchdunger, E., Ohno, S., Segal, G. M., Fanning, S., et al. Effects of a selective inhibitor of the Abl tyrosine kinase on the growth of Bcr-Abl positive cells. *Nat. Med.* [Research Support, Non-US Gov't Research Support, US Gov't, P.H.S.]. 1996 May;2(5):561-6.
[67] Deininger, M. W., Goldman, J. M., Lydon, N., Melo, J. V. The tyrosine kinase inhibitor CGP57148B selectively inhibits the growth of BCR-ABL-positive cells. *Blood.* [Research Support, Non-US Gov't]. 1997 Nov. 1;90(9):3691-8.
[68] Barak, A. F., Bonstein, L., Lauterbach, R., Naparstek, E., Tavor, S. Tyrosine kinase inhibitors induced immune thrombocytopenia in chronic myeloid leukemia? *Hematol. Rep.* 2011 Oct. 19;3(3):e29.
[69] Mattiuzzi, G. N., Cortes, J. E., Talpaz, M., Reuben, J., Rios, M. B., Shan, J., et al. Development of Varicella-Zoster virus infection in patients with chronic myelogenous leukemia treated with imatinib mesylate. *Clin. Cancer Res.* 2003 Mar.;9(3):976-80.
[70] Atallah, E., Durand, J. B., Kantarjian, H., Cortes, J. Congestive heart failure is a rare event in patients receiving imatinib therapy. *Blood.* 2007 Aug. 15;110(4):1233-7.
[71] Kerkela, R., Grazette, L., Yacobi, R., Iliescu, C., Patten, R., Beahm, C., et al. Cardiotoxicity of the cancer therapeutic agent imatinib mesylate. *Nat. Med.* 2006 Aug.; 12(8):908-16.
[72] Garcia-Alvarez, A., Sitges, M., Garcia-Albeniz, X., Sionis, A., Loma-Osorio, P., Bosch, X. Atypical cardiac manifestation of hypereosinophilic syndrome and reversible cardiotoxicity to imatinib. *Int. J. Cardiol.* 2010 Mar. 4;139(2):e29-31.
[73] Steegmann, J. L., Cervantes, F., le Coutre, P., Porkka, K., Saglio, G. Off-target effects of BCR-ABL1 inhibitors and their potential long-term implications in patients with chronic myeloid leukemia. *Leuk. Lymphoma.* 2012 Jun. 18.
[74] Cohen, M. H., Williams, G., Johnson, J. R., Duan, J., Gobburu, J., Rahman, A., et al. Approval summary for imatinib mesylate capsules in the treatment of chronic myelogenous leukemia. *Clin. Cancer Res.* 2002 May;8(5):935-42.
[75] Quintas-Cardama, A., Cortes, J. E., Kantarjian, H. Practical management of toxicities associated with tyrosine kinase inhibitors in chronic myeloid leukemia. *Clin. Lymphoma Myeloma.* [Research Support, Non-US Gov't Review]. 2008 Mar.;8 Suppl. 3:S82-8.
[76] Marcolino, M. S., Boersma, E., Clementino, N. C., Macedo, A. V., Marx-Neto, A. D., Silva, M. H., et al. Imatinib treatment duration is related to decreased estimated

glomerular filtration rate in chronic myeloid leukemia patients. *Ann. Oncol.* 2011 Sep.; 22(9):2073-9.

[77] Ozkurt, S., Temiz, G., Acikalin, M. F., Soydan, M. Acute renal failure under dasatinib therapy. *Ren. Fail.* [Case Reports Review]. 2010 Jan.;32(1):147-9.

[78] Berman, E., Nicolaides, M., Maki, R. G., Fleisher, M., Chanel, S., Scheu, K., et al. Altered bone and mineral metabolism in patients receiving imatinib mesylate. *N Engl. J. Med.* 2006 May 11;354(19):2006-13.

[79] Zekri, J. M., Robinson, M. H., Woll, P. J. Relative hypocalcaemia and muscle cramps in patients receiving imatinib for gastrointestinal stromal tumour. *Sarcoma.* 2006;2006 (1):48948.

[80] Gordon, J. K., Magid, S. K., Maki, R. G., Fleisher, M., Berman, E. Elevations of creatine kinase in patients treated with imatinib mesylate (Gleevec). *Leuk. Res.* 2010 Jun.;34(6):827-9.

[81] Van Oosterom, A. T., Judson, I., Verweij, J., Stroobants, S., Donato di Paola, E., Dimitrijevic, S., et al. Safety and efficacy of imatinib (STI571) in metastatic gastrointestinal stromal tumours: a phase I study. *Lancet.* 2001 Oct. 27;358(9291): 1421-3.

[82] Etienne, G., Cony-Makhoul, P., Mahon, F. X. Imatinib mesylate and gray hair. *N Engl. J. Med.* 2002 Aug. 8;347(6):446.

[83] Brouard, M. C., Prins, C., Mach-Pascual, S., Saurat, J. H. Acute generalized exanthematous pustulosis associated with STI571 in a patient with chronic myeloid leukemia. *Dermatology.* 2001;203(1):57-9.

[84] Hsiao, L. T., Chung, H. M., Lin, J. T., Chiou, T. J., Liu, J. H., Fan, F. S., et al. Stevens-Johnson syndrome after treatment with STI571: a case report. *Br. J. Haematol.* 2002 Jun.;117(3):620-2.

[85] Kim, T. D., Schwarz, M., Nogai, H., Grille, P., Westermann, J., Plockinger, U., et al. Thyroid dysfunction caused by second-generation tyrosine kinase inhibitors in Philadelphia chromosome-positive chronic myeloid leukemia. *Thyroid.* 2010 Nov.;20 (11):1209-14.

[86] De Groot, J. W., Zonnenberg, B. A., Plukker, J. T., van Der Graaf, W. T., Links, T. P. Imatinib induces hypothyroidism in patients receiving levothyroxine. *Clin. Pharmacol. Ther.* 2005 Oct.;78(4):433-8.

[87] Gambacorti-Passerini, C., Tornaghi, L., Cavagnini, F., Rossi, P., Pecori-Giraldi, F., Mariani, L., et al. Gynaecomastia in men with chronic myeloid leukaemia after imatinib. *Lancet.* 2003 Jun. 7;361(9373):1954-6.

[88] Seshadri, T., Seymour, J. F., McArthur, G. A. Oligospermia in a patient receiving imatinib therapy for the hypereosinophilic syndrome. *N Engl. J. Med.* 2004 Nov. 11; 351(20):2134-5.

[89] Christopoulos, C., Dimakopoulou, V., Rotas, E. Primary ovarian insufficiency associated with imatinib therapy. *N Engl. J. Med.* 2008 Mar. 6;358(10):1079-80.

[90] Duman, B. B., Paydas, S., Disel, U., Besen, A., Gurkan, E. Secondary malignancy after imatinib therapy: eight cases and review of the literature. *Leuk. Lymphoma.* 2012 Apr. 2.

[91] Verma, D., Kantarjian, H., Strom, S. S., Rios, M. B., Jabbour, E., Quintas-Cardama, A., et al. Malignancies occurring during therapy with tyrosine kinase inhibitors (TKIs) for

chronic myeloid leukemia (CML) and other hematologic malignancies. *Blood.* [Research Support, N.I.H., Extramural]. 2011 Oct. 20;118(16):4353-8.

[92] Millot, F., Baruchel, A., Guilhot, J., Petit, A., Leblanc, T., Bertrand, Y., et al. Imatinib is effective in children with previously untreated chronic myelogenous leukemia in early chronic phase: results of the French national phase IV trial. *J. Clin. Oncol.* 2011 Jul. 10;29(20):2827-32.

[93] Kieswetter, K., Schwartz, Z., Alderete, M., Dean, D. D., Boyan, B. D. Platelet derived growth factor stimulates chondrocyte proliferation but prevents endochondral maturation. *Endocrine.* [Comparative Study]. 1997 Jun.;6(3):257-64.

[94] Rastogi, M. V., Stork, L., Druker, B., Blasdel, C., Nguyen, T., Boston, B. A. Imatinib mesylate causes growth deceleration in pediatric patients with chronic myelogenous leukemia. *Pediatr. Blood Cancer.* 2012 Feb. 29.

[95] Hensley, M. L., Ford, J. M. Imatinib treatment: specific issues related to safety, fertility, and pregnancy. *Semin. Hematol.* 2003 Apr.;40(2 Suppl. 2):21-5.

[96] Ault, P., Kantarjian, H., O'Brien, S., Faderl, S., Beran, M., Rios, M. B., et al. Pregnancy among patients with chronic myeloid leukemia treated with imatinib. *J. Clin. Oncol.* 2006 Mar. 1;24(7):1204-8.

[97] Ramasamy, K., Hayden, J., Lim, Z., Mufti, G. J., Ho, A. Y. Successful pregnancies involving men with chronic myeloid leukaemia on imatinib therapy. *Br. J. Haematol.* 2007 May;137(4):374-5.

In: Imatinib
Editors: Mojtaba Akhtari and Ihab Elhemaidi
ISBN: 978-1-62808-297-5

Chapter 4

Practical Approach to the Hematologic Adverse Effects of Imatinib

Mojbata Akhtari*[*] *and Nicholas A. Barber
Division of Hematology and Oncology, Department of Internal Medicine,
Nebraska Medical Center, University of Nebraska Medical Center, Omaha, US

Introduction

Originally developed for CML, imatinib mesylate (Gleevec®, Novartis, East Hanover, NJ) is approved for multiple hematologic and solid malignancies (Table 1) [1]. In addition to BCR-ABL imatinib also inhibits the c-kit, platelet derived growth factor *(PDGF),* and other molecular pathways responsible for tumorgenesis. Before the approval of imatinib in 2001 the prognosis of patients with CML was poor (average survival of 3-7 years) [2]. Since the introduction of imatinib the 8-year survival is now greater than 85% [3].

Table 1. Imatinib: FDA Approved Indications and Dosing

Indication	Dose (mg/day)
Adult Ph+ CML CP	400
Adult Ph+ CML AP or BC	600
Pediatric Ph+ CML	340 /m^2
Adult Ph+ ALL	600
Adult MDS/MPD	400
Adults agressive systemic mastocytosis	100 or 400
Aduld hypereosinophilic syndrome of chronic eosinophilic leukemia	100 or 400
Adult dermatofibrosarcoma protuberans	800
Adults metastatic or unresectable GIST	400

[*] Email: Mojtaba.akhtari@unmc.edu.

Table 1. (Continued)

Indication	Dose (mg/day)
Adult adjuvant GIST	400
Gleevec package insert. Used with permission	

Cytopenias

Imatinib-induced cytopenias are most commonly seen in patients with CML but can also be seen in patients treated for other diseases. Cytopenias are more common in those who have received prior cytotoxic therapy and in those with advanced phases of CML.

Etiology

The etiology of imatinib-induced cytopenias in patients with CML may be explained by a number of mechanisms. Cytopenias develop acutely during therapeutic elimination of leukemic marrow cells resulting in a transientl hypocellular marrow that exists until normal hematopoiesis resumes. This is the most likely explanation for the more severe cytopenias seen in advanced staged CML. This phenomenon has been confirmed by interim marrow analysis of patients recently started on imatinib [4-6]. One of these reports involved an analysis of bone marrow samples of 52 patients receiving imatinib in multiple phase II studies. The investigators reported a decrease in cellularity to ≤ 50% in 41 (77%) of these patients. This also supports the fact that there is a decreasing incidence of cytopenias over time and as patients have achieved remission.

Also contributing to myelosuppression is direct inhibition of multiple tyrosine kinase pathways that promote normal hematopoiesis. Specifically, inhibition of the c-Abl pathway causes cell-cycle arrest and prevents normal differentiation of CD34+ cells [7-9]. The inhibition of c-Kit may explain why a small number of patients treated with imatinib for GIST who have normal baseline marrow function develop cytopenias (grade 3 or 4 neutropenia 5%, anemia 2%) [10]. The c-Kit pathway may play a larger role than PDGFR in maintaining normal hematopoiesis. This may explain why patients with hypereosinophilic syndrome as well as chronic myelomonocytic leukemia (CMML) and the rearranged PDGFRß gene who are treated with imatinib do not experience significant cytopenias [11-12].

Clinical Trial Data for CML

Table 2 summarizes the incidences of imatinib-induced cytopenias in the various phase II and phase III trials that have led to drug approval.

Table 2. Summary of Grade 3 or 4 cytopenias in clinical trials of imatinib

Trial		Dose	Neutropenia (%)	Anemia (%)	Thrombocytopenia (%)
Kantarjian, et al [13]	Phase II, late CML after failure of interferon	400 mg daily	35	7	20
O'Brien, et al [14,15]	Phase III imatinib vs. interferon plus low dose cytarabine for newly diagnosed CP CML (IRIS)	400 mg daily	14	3	8
Talpaz, et al [16]	Phase II AP CML	400 or 600 mg daily	56 (400 mg), 60 (600 mg)	44 (400 mg), 47 (600 mg)	44 (400 mg), 43 (600 mg)
Sawyers, et al [17]	Phase II BP CML	600 mg daily	64	62	52
Demetri, et al [10]	Phase II advanced GIST	400 or 600 mg daily	6.8 (400 mg), 2.1 (600 mg)	1.4 (400), 2.7 (600 mg)	NR
Verweiji, et al [18]	Phase II advanced GIST	400 mg daily or bid	7 (400 mg daily), 7 (400 mg bid)	7 (400 mg daily), 17 (400 mg bid)	1.4 (400 mg daily), 1.3 (400 mg bid)

Patients Who Have Received Prior Therapy

Grade 3 or 4 cytopenias are more common in patients with prior exposure to chemotherapy and cytokine therapy. This is illustrated by a number of trials including the original phase II trial of imatinib for late CP CML after interferon alpha failure [13]. In this trial grade 3 or 4 cytopenias were seen frequently: neutropenia (35%), thrombocytopenia (20%), and anemia (7%). Median time-to-develop and duration of grade 3 or 4 neutropenic or thrombocytopenic episodes were 62 days (duration 21 days) and 57 days (duration 18 days) respectively. Patients with pre-existing anemia and prior hydroxyurea, interferon, and busulfan experience more myelosuppression [19].

Despite this high initial rate of cytopenias that often required treatment modifications and interruptions, the incidence significantly decreased after one year of therapy. A six-year follow-up of this trial compared rates of cytopenias during and after the first year of imatinib therapy [20]. Grade 3 or 4 neutropenia was less than half as frequent (13%) during subsequent years of therapy and was less than 1% after two years. Although gradual reconstitution of the marrow with healthy hematopoietic progenitor cells may partially explain this, a significant decrease in the incidence of cytopenias can be explained by the dropout of patients with disease progression [19].

To further illustrate the increased rate of cytopenias in patients with prior exposure to therapy, Breccia et al compared toxicities of patients treated in early or late (after failure of interferon) CP CML and found that grade 3 or 4 cytopenias were seen in 7% and 24% of patients respectively [21]. They also found shorter median duration of cytopenias in early CP CML (10-14 days) compared to LP CML (16-20 days).

Disease Phase and Dose Dependence

The severity of cytopenias correlates with disease phase. A phase II trial of imatinib in 229 patients with BP CML reported grade 3-4 neutropenia (64%), thrombocytopenia (62%), and anemia (52%) [17]. In this study, the median days to reach a thrombocytopenic and neutropenic nadir were 37 and 36 respectively. Median days to recovery were 31 for thrombocytopenia and 19 for neutropenia. This report did not include a description of therapy received prior to imatinib but did report a median of over three years since diagnosis. Another phase II study involving 181 pre-treated patients with AP CML (including 29 patients in BP) reported higher rates of grade 3 or 4 cytopenias with two different doses of imatinib: neutropenia (56% with 400 mg, 60% with 600 mg), thrombocytopenia (44% with 400 mg, 43% with 600 mg), and anemia (44% with 400 mg, 47% with 600 mg) [16].

Dose dependence was also illustrated by a phase III trial compared 800 mg daily to 400 mg daily in patients with pre-treated CML [22]. The authors reported almost twice the incidence of grade 3 or 4 cytopenias in the higher dose group: leukopenia (46% vs 24%), anemia (14% vs 2%), and thrombocytopenia (39% vs 15%).

Upfront and Chemotherapy Naïve

In contrast, cytopenias are much less frequent in patients receiving imatinib as upfront therapy for newly diagnosed CP CML. This is illustrated by the results from the IRIS study [14-15]. This trial randomized over 1,000 patients with newly diagnosed chronic phase (CP) CML to either imatinib 400 mg daily or a combination of interferon alpha and cytarabine. The overall frequency of grade 3 or 4 cytopenias with imatinib was much less than the chemotherapy arm: neutropenia (14.3% vs 25%), thrombocytopenia (7.8% vs 16.5%), and anemia (3.1% vs 4.3%) respectively. Similar to earlier experience, the majority of cytopenias were seen within the first two years with grade 3 or 4 cytopenias reported in < 5% of patients after two years.

Neutropenic Fever

Although the phase II BP CML trial reported neutropenic fever or severe sepsis in 6-17% of patients, it is uncommon in CP CML (less than 1%) [13,17,23]. In the initial phase II study of late CP CML after failure of interferon, neutropenic fever was reported in only 0.75% of patients. The virtual absence of mucositis as a side effect of imatinib is the most likely explanation for this.

Drug Discontinuation and Dose Modifications

Hematologic intolerance to imatinib leading to dose modifications, treatment delays, and therapeutic substitutions with newer generation TKIs are not uncommon. Most of the time myelosuppression is the cause. In the IRIS study only 2% of patients discontinued imatinib because of drug related adverse events [24].

In an ASCO abstract presented in 2007 Hamden et al analyzed dosing trends for 216 patients who were receiving imatinib for CML (87% in CP) between 2000-2005 [25]. Dose reductions were required in 21%, 59%, and 67% of patients taking 400 mg, 600 mg, and 800 mg respectively. Most common reasons for dose reduction were grade 3 to 4 cytopenias. Treatment was suspended in 29% of patients, most commonly for persistent anemia and thrombocytopenia. After holding imatinib for a median of 21 days, 74% of these patients were able to resume therapy while the remaining 26% permanently discontinued the drug.

Clinical Significance of Therapy Related Cytopenias

Patients, who develop cytopenias, and particularly those who require dose reductions or interruptions, tend to have worse outcomes. This is illustrated by a follow-up analysis of the original phase II study of imatinib after interferon failure.[26] In this study, the authors showed that the presence of imatinib-induced neutropenia (<1,000 neutrophils/mm^3) at three months after the initiation of therapy, along with a poor cytogenetic response, are independent predictive factor for blast transformation and decreased survival. A follow-up of the original phase II study of imatinib in patients who failed interferon found that any episode of grade 3 or 4 myelosuppression, especially those that lasted longer than two weeks, was associated with lower rates of major (58% vs 75%) and complete (36% and 63%) cytogenetic responses [27].

Table 3. Correlation between occurrence of hematological toxicity in a period less than 6 months or at more than 12 months from the onset of imatinib and absence of CCR

		No. of patients that did not achieve CCR/No. of patients experienced hematological toxicity (%)	
	Grade of toxicity	Toxicity occurring less than 6 months after onset of imatinib	Toxicity occurring at more than 12 months after onset of imatinib
Late CP patients	1	6/20 (30)	6/20 (30)
	2	15/25 (60)	11/25 (44)
	3 to 4	8/14 (57)	8/14 (57)
Early CP patients	1	7/11 (63)*	3/11 (27)*
	2	9/13 (69)*	4/11 (36)*
	3 to 4	2/2 (100)*	1/2 (50)*
*p = 0.001.			
CCR, complete cytogenetic response; CP, chronic phase. Used with permission. [21]			

Treatment delays and discontinuation as a result of severe myelosuppression and a greater tumor burden at the initiation of treatment are both implicated in these unfavorable outcomes. It is important to understand that this analysis was done on patients with more advanced disease (late CP CML and prior interferon therapy) rather than early CP CML where major cytogenetic responses were shown to be significantly higher (85% vs 60%) [14, 13].

In addition to studying the differences of imatinib-induced cytopenias in early and late CP-CML Breccia et al also correlated these with disease response [21]. Grade 3 to 4 cytopenias were more common in patients with late CP CML (24 % vs 7 %, $p = 0.0001$). Dose interruptions and reductions in late (19% and 6%) and early (14% and 12%) CP CML respectively. Although the study compared small numbers of patients, they found that only the early CP CML patients who experienced cytopenias of any grade within the first six months of therapy achieved significantly fewer complete cytogenetic responses (Table 3). This is contrasted to the apparent favorable predictor of imatinib induced reduction of marrow cellularity, which will be discussed below.

Recommended Management of Imatinb-Induced Myelosuppression

Recommendations for Monitoring and Therapy Modification

Guidelines for monitoring imatinib induced cytopenias have been well described [28-29]. A panel of experts recommends that complete blood counts be done weekly for the first month, monthly during month 2 and 3, and every three months thereafter. The package insert for imatinib recommends checking complete blood counts weekly for the first month, biweekly for the second month, and as clinically indicated therafter [1].

Table 4. NCCN Guidelines for the Management of Imatinib-Induced Cytopenias [30]

	Imatinib	
Neutropenia	Thrombocytopenia	Patients with AP/BP
Hold until ANC $\geq$ 1500/mm^3, then resume at the starting dose of 400 mg. If recurrence of ANC < 1000/mm^3, hold until ANC $\geq$ 1500/mm^3, then resume at reduced dose of 300 mg	Hold until Plt $\geq$ 75,000/mm^3, then resume at starting dose of 400 mg. If recurrence of plt < 50,000/mm^3, hold until plt $\geq$ 75,000/mm^3, then resume at reduced dose of 300 mg.	Rule out disease related cytopenias. If not related to disease, reduce dose to 400 mg. if cytopenia persists 2 weeks, reduce dose further to 300 mg. If cytopenias persist for 4 weeks, stop imatinib until ANC $\geq$ 1000/mm^3 and platelet count $\geq$ 20,000/mm^3, and then resume treatment at 300 mg.

Guidelines for the management of imatinib-induced cytopenias have been established by a number of institutions including the FDA and the National Comprehensive Cancer Network (NCCN) (Table 4) [1, 19, 30]. A number of important concepts apply when considering therapy modification:

1. More aggressive disease should afford greater tolerance for hematologic toxicities in order to avoid treatment disruptions
2. Neutropenic complications are rare in imatinib-induced neutropenia
3. Blood products and myeloid growth factor support is generally encouraged in higher risk patients
4. Grade 1 or 2 myelosuppression does not require modification of therapy
5. Intolerance to one BCR-ABL TKI agent merits a trial with another
6. Bone marrow biopsy should be considered if the clinician suspects that cytopenias are due to disease response rather than drug toxicity. Differentiating the cause may improve long-term outcomes [27].

The Role of Hematopoietic Growth Factors

Because therapy interruptions and dose modifications have been associated with less favorable outcomes, the use of hematopoetic stimulating agents has been suggested.

The rationale for using granulocyte-colony stimulating factor (G-CSF) is to avoid infectious complications and to allow for uninterrupted therapy and the achievement of remission. Improvement in imatinib-induced neutropenia through the use of filgrastim has been reported [31]. Most patients in this series experienced improved hematologic tolerance leading to increased adherence. The authors also observed that after filgrastim was given more patients achieved cytogenetic responses. Martin et al described 11 patients with either CP or AP CML who had failed to achieve a cytogenetic response six months after starting imatinib and who required interruption of therapy due to grade 3 to 4 neutropenia [32]. All patients were re-challenged with imatinib at 300 mg daily along with filgrastim 300 micrograms 2-3 times per week. After starting filgrastim seven (64%) of these patients achieved major cytogenetic response (1 complete cytogenetic response) within 6-12 months. Another series suggests that G-CSF may improve disease outcomes by stimulating 'dormant', but otherwise TKI resistant, leukemic cells into a susceptible state [33]. The guidelines by Mauro et al include G-CSF as an option in the management of imatinib-induced neutropenia [19].

The presence of anemia during imatinib therapy may be associated with a lower probability of complete cytogenetic response as well as inferior survival [34]. The use of erythropoietin stimulating agents (ESA) has been investigated as a means to overcome this [35]. In a cohort of 608 patients with CP CML the use of ESAs was reviewed along with the achievement of cytogenetic response and survival. In this study 217 patients required ESAs for anemia. The authors confirmed that severe anemia was associated with worse outcomes but that the use of ESAs did not improve either cytogenetic response rate or survival. Throbotic complications were higher in patients receiving ESAs.

Reduction in Bone Marrow Cellularity

Most patients who develop cytopenias from imatinib recover within two months of dose reduction or discontinuation. However, a number of bone marrow changes have been described.

Table 5. Correlation of bone marrow morphologic features with cytogenetic response to STI571 therapy*

	Patients with observed change	Patients with cytogenetic response (<65% Ph+)	Correlation of change with cytogenetic response**
Decrease in cellularity	41/53 (77)	17/41 (41)	P = 0.04
Development of severe hypoplasia	7/53 (13)	2/7 (29)	P > 1.99
Development of erythroid hyperplasia	34/53 (64)	13/34 (38)	P = 0.55
Resolution of reticulin fibrosis	15/21 (71)	4/15 (27)	P = 0.61
Reduction in megakaryocyte number and clustering	19/34 (56)	8/19 (42)	P = 0.45
Normalization of megakaryocyte morphologic features	17/35 (49)	5/17 (29)	P = 0.49
All patients		18/53 (34)	
Ph+, Philadelphia chromosome - positive			
* Data are given as number of patients with the change or response/number of patients assessed (%). Definitions of changes in features are as follows: decreased cellularity, 50% or less cellularity; severe hypoplasia, 5% or less cellularity; erythroid hyperplasia, myeloid/erythroid ratio of 1 or less; resolution of reticulin fibrosis, decrease of at least 2 grades; reduction in megakaryocyte number and clustering, <15mm2 and lack of clusters; normalization of megakaryocyte morphologic features, <25% forms with monolobate nuclei.			
**Fisher exact test			
[36]			

Imatinib can reduce overall marrow cellularity and has been well described in a series of 53 patients who underwent bone marrow examination during therapy to specifically assess treatment effects [36].

This series included patients in all phases of CML (20 CP, 16 AP, and 17 BP) and in those who had received prior chemotherapy. A greater than 50% decrease in marrow cellularity was seen in 77% of patients. Further characterizations of bone marrow changes including reticulin fibrosis and reduction in megakaryocytes as well as correlation with disease response are shown in table 5.

Interestingly, patients who developed at least 50% reduction in marrow cellularity had a significantly higher cytogenetic response (94% of all patients achieving a cytogenetic response of < 65% Ph+; $P = 0.04$). This series did not correlate marrow cellularity with peripheral blood counts.

Other Bone Marrow Disorders

Bone Marrow Aplasia

Bone marrow aplasia (BMA) has been well described in patients treated in all phases of CML [37-38]. Srinvas et al reported the largest series of 44 patients treated in various phases of CML who underwent bone marrow biopsy to evaluate persistent pancytopenia that developed after three to six months of imatinib. Five patients (two in CP, two in BP, and one in AP) had BMA (5-10% cellularity). The three patients who were in CP or AP developed aplasia after six months of therapy and at doses of 400 mg daily and 600 mg daily respectively. In contrast the two patients treated in BP developed aplasia only after three months of therapy and at doses of 800 mg daily. One of these patients died of an intracranial hemorrhage. All five patients were positive for BCR-ABL RT-PCR at the time of marrow analysis. This is consistent with the fact that patients who develop more severe cytopenias achieve remissions less frequently. Histories of prior chemotherapy in all five patients as well as long-term follow up on the remaining four patients were not included. Some patients who develop severe BMA can be transfusion dependent for months and one fatal case has been reported in a woman with prior busulfan and interferon exposure [39].

Gelatinous Marrow Transformation

Gelatinous marrow transformation (GMT) is characterized by adipocyte atrophy, hematopoietic cell hypoplasia, and deposition of hyaluronic acid (HA) extracellular matrix. It is a rare manifestation of hematologic malignancies as well and non-malignant diseases such as alcoholism and chronic infections [40]. The diagnosis is established by bone marrow staining positive for the HA binding chemical Alcian blue. A handful of cases of GMT in patients taking imatinib for CML have been reported [40-41]. All three reported patients had received imatinib as initial therapy for CP CML and developed persistent cytopenias leading to bone marrow biopsy. GMT led to a dose reduction in one patient; a decision to pursue a matched related donor allotransplant in the second patient; and a switch to nilotinib in the third patient. In these patients, the presence of GMT did not portend a worse prognosis. The mechanism for this process is not well understood but may be secondary to leukemic cell production of hyaluronic acid or direct bone marrow stroma toxicity (i.e. imatinib).

Bone Marrow Necrosis

Multiple cases of bone marrow necrosis (BMN) have been reported in patients taking imatinib for CML and Ph+ ALL [42-43]. BMN has been reported in CML patients before the development of imatinib which suggests a TKI-independent mechanism [44-45]. In addition, three cases of bone marrow necrosis (two involving the pelvis and one involving the thoracic vertebrae) have been reported in patients treated with imatinib for metastatic GIST [46-47]. All three patients had achieved good systemic responses to imatinib making the existence of new osseous metastasis unlikely. This led to bone biopsies that confirmed the diagnosis of BMN. One patient underwent vertebral corpectomy due to concern for spinal instability.

Hemolytic Anemia

Rare cases of both Coombs' positive and negative autoimmune hemolysis have been reported in patients taking imatinib [48-49]. A patient who developed Coomb's positive disease had imatinib-specific antibodies confirmed on gel microcolumn assay. The Coombs' negative patient was being treated for GIST and also developed a drug-induced maculopapular rash. Both reported patients responded to steroids and were able to resume imatinib.

Thrombotic Thrombocytopenic Purpura

Thrombotic thrombocytopenic purpura (TTP) associated with imatinib has also been reported in a patient with idiopathic hypereosinophilic syndrome [50]. This patient had initially received steroids, hydroxyurea, and allopurinol for the hypereosinophilia but did not repond. Imatinib 400 mg daily was started but was stopped after five days because the patient developed acute renal failure, thrombocytopenia, and microangiopathic hemolysis. A renal biopsy as well as a suppressed ADAMTS-13 level confirmed the diagnosis of TTP. The patient eventually recovered from TTP after undergoing plasma exchange. Interestingly, the hypereosinophilia resolved without the need for further therapy.

Macrocytosis

Macrocytosis has been reported in up to 42% of patients taking imatinib for advanced GIST [51-53]. In one series, all patients developed macrocytosis with mean corpuscular volume (MCV) increases of 0.7%, 5.6%, 5.9%, and 5% after 3, 6, 9, and 12 months of therapy respectively. There did not appear to be any adverse outcomes in patients who developed an increased MCV. Inhibition of c-kit, and perhaps other pathways promoting erythroid differentiation are the proposed mechanism for this phenomenon. Macrocytosis resolved after imatinib was discontinued.

Conclusion

The most common hematologic toxicities of imatinib are cytopenias. Cytopenias are commonly seen in CML but can also be seen in advanced GIST. Cytopenias may develop due to either direct myelosuppression or eradication of a hypercellular marrow lacking healthy Philadelphia-negative hematopoietic precursors. The severities of cytopenias typically correlate with dosage, disease burden, prior cytotoxic or cytokine therapy, and advanced phases of disease. Neutropenic fever is infrequent because patients do not get mucositis.

Imatinib-induced cytopenias have also been associated with worse disease outcomes in CML, likely due to treatment delays. Myeloid growth factor administration may improve treatment continuity and outcomes whereas erythropoietic stimulating agents do not improve outcomes but do increase thrombotic complications. Frequent upfront monitoring for cytopenias is recommended until complete blood count stability is observed. Management guidelines for TKI-induced cytopenias, including myeloid growth factor administration, are well established. Although a reduction in bone marrow cellularity is associated with better disease response, prolonged bone marrow aplasia, bone marrow necrosis, and gelatinous marrow transformation are rarely found to cause prolonged cytopenias and may adversely affect continuity of therapy. Other less common hematologic problems associated with imatinib include hemolytic anemia and TTP. Macrocytosis without nutritional deficiency has been well described with imatinib, especially in patients with advanced GIST.

References

[1] Prescribing information. Gleevec®(imatinib mesylate) Novartis Pharmaceuticals Corporation. East Hanover, NJ. Revised 04/2011.

[2] Sawyers CL (1999). Chronic Myeloid Leukemia. *N. Engl. J. Med.,* 340:1330-1340.

[3] Deininger M, O'Brien SG, Guilhot F, Goldman JM, Hochhaus A, Hughes TP, Radich JP, Hatfield AK, Mone M, Filian J, Reynolds J, Gathmann I, Larson RA, Druker BJ (2009). International randomized study of interferon Vs ST1571 (IRIS) 8-year follow up: sustained survival and low risk for progression or events in patients with newly diagnosed chronic myeloid leukemia in chronic phas (CML-CP) treated with imatinib. ASCO Abstract 1126.

[4] Mauro MJ, Deininger MW (2009). Management of drug toxicities in chronic myeloid leukaemia. *B Pract. & Res. Clin. Haem.,* 22:409-429.

[5] Paul TR, Uppin SG, Uppin MS, Jacob RT, Rao DR, Rajappa SJ (2010). Evaluation of cytopenias occurring in imatinib treated chronic myeloid leukemia (CML) patients. *Indian J. Hematol. Blood Transfus.,* 26:56-61.

[6] Hasserjian RP, Boecklin F, Parker S, Chase A, Dhar S, Zaiac M, Olavarria E, Lampert I, Henry K, Apperley JF, Goldman JM (2002) STI571 (Imatinib Mesylate) reduces bone marrow cellularity and normalizes morphologic features irrespective of cytogenetic response. *Hematopathology,* 117:360-367.

[7] Rosti V, Bergamaschi G, Lucotti C, Danova M, Carlo-Stella C, Localetti F, Tonon L, Mazzini G, Cazzola M (1995) Oligodeoxynucleotides antisense to c-abl specifically inhibit entry.

[8] Brandt j, Briddell RA, Srour EF, Leemhuis TB, Hoffman R (1992). Role of c-kit ligand in the expansion of human hematopoietic progenitor cells. *Blood,* 79:634-641.

[9] Su RJ, Zhang XB, Li K, Yang M, Li CK, Fok TF, James AE, Pong H, Yuen PM (2002). Platelet-derived growth factor promotes ex vivo expansion of CD34+ cells from human cord blood and enhances long-term culture-initiating cells, non-obese diabetic/severe combined immunodeficient repopulating cells and formation of adherent cells. *Br. J. Haematol.,* 117:735-746.

[10] Demetri GD, von Mehren M, Blanke CD, Van Den Abbeele AD, Eisenberg B, Roberts PJ, Heinrich MC, Tuveson DA, Singer S, Janicek M, Fletcher JA, Silverman SG, Silberman SL, Capdeville R, Kiese B, Peng B, Dimitrijevic S, Druker BJ, Corless C, Fletcher CDM, Joensuu H (2002). Efficacy and safety of imatinib mesylate in advanced gastrointestinal stromal tumors. *N. Engl. J. Med.,* 347: 472-480.

[11] Pardanani A, Reeder T, Porrata LF, Li CY, Tazelaar HD, Baxter EJ, Witzig TE, Cross NCP, Tefferi A (2003). Imatinib therapy for hypereosinophilic syndrome and other eosinophilic disorders. *Blood,* 101:3391-3397.

[12] Galimberti S, Ferreri MI, Simi P, Azzara A, Barate C, Fazzi R, Cecconi N, Cervetti G, Guerrini F, Petrini M (2009). Platelet-derived growth factor beta receptor (*PDGFRB*) gene is rearranged in a significant percentage of myelodysplastic syndromes with normal karyotype. *Brit. J. Haem.,* 147:760-774.

[13] Kantarjian H, Sawyers C, Hochhaus A, Guilhot F, Schiffer C, Gambocorti-Passerini C, Niederwieser D, Resta D, Capdeville R, Zoellner U, Talpaz M, Druker B (2002). Hematologic and cytogenetic responses to imatinib mesylate in chronic myelogenous leukemia. *N. Engl. J. Med.,* 346: 645-652.

[14] O'Brien S, Guilhot F, Larson R, Gathmann I, Baccarani M, Cervantes F, Cornelissen JJ, Fischer T, Hochhaus A, Hughes T, Lechner K, Nielsen JL, Rousselot P, Reiffers J, Saglio G, Shepherd J, Simonsson B, Gratwohl A, Goldman JM, Kantarjian H, Taylor K, Verhoef G, Bolton AE, Capdeville R, Druker BJ (2003). Imatinib compared with interferon and low-dose cytarabine for newly diagnosed chronic-phase chronic myeloid leukemia. *N. Engl. J. Med.,* 348:994-1004.

[15] Druker BJ, Guilhot F, O'Brien SG, Gathmann I, Kantarjian H, Gattermann N, Deininger MW, Silver RT, Goldman JM, Stone RM, Gervantes F, Hochhaus A, Powell BL, Gabrilove JL, Rousselot P, Reiffers J, Corelissen JJ, Hughes T, Agis H, Fischer T, Verhoef G, Shepherd J, Saglio G, Gratwohl A, Nielsen JL, Radich JP, Simonsson B, Taylor K, Baccarani M, So C, Letvak L, Larson R (2006). Five-year follow-up of patients receiving imatinib for chronic myeloid leukemia. *N. Engl. J. Med.,* 355:2408-2417.

[16] Talpaz M, Silver RT, Druker BJ, Goldman JM, Gambacorti-Passerini C, Guilhot F, Schiffer CA, Fischer T, Deininger MWN, Lennard AL, Hochhaus A, Ottmann OG, Gratwohl A, Baccarani M, Stone R, Tura S, Mahon FX, Fernandes-Reese S, Gathmann I, Capdeville R, Kantarjian HM, Sawyers (2002). Imatinib induces durable hematologic and cytogentetic responses in patients with accelerated phase chronic myeloid leukemia: results of a phase 2 study. *Blood,* 99: 1928-1937.

[17] Sawyers CL, Hochhaus A, Feldman E, Goldman JM, Miller CB, Ottmann OG, Schiffer CA, Talpaz M, Guilhot F, Deininger MWN, Fischer T, O'Brien SG, Stone RM, Gambacorti-Passerini CB, Russell NH, Reiffers JJ, Shea TC, Chapuis B, Courtre S, Tura S, Morra E, Larson RA, Saven A, Peschel C, Gratwohl A, Mandelli F, Ben-Am M, Gathmann I, Capdeville R, Paquette RL, Druker BJ (2002). Imatinib induces hematologic and cytogenetic responses in patients with chronic myelogenous leukemia in myeloid blast crisis: results of a phase II study: presented in part at the 43rd Annual meeting of the American Society of Hematology, Orlando, FL, December 11, 2001. *Blood,* 99:3530-3539.

[18] Verweij J, Casali PG, Zalcberg J, LeCesne A, Reichardt P, Blay JY, Issels R, van Oosterom A, Hogendoom PCW, Van Glabbeke M, Bertulli R, Judson (2004).

Progression-free survival in gastrointestinal stromal tumours with high-dose imatinib: randomized trial. *Lancet,* 364:1127-1134.

[19] Mauro MJ, Deininger MW (2009). Management of drug toxicities in chronic myeloid leukaemia. *B Pract. & Res. Clin. Haem.,* 22:409-429.

[20] Hochhaus A, Druker B, Sawyers C, Guilhot F, Schiffer CA, Cortes J, Niederwieser DW, Gambacorti-Passerini C, Stone RM, Goldman J, Fischer T, O'Brien SG, Reiffers JJ, Mone M, Krahnke T, Talpaz M, Kantarjian HM (2008). Favorable long-term follow-up results over 6 years for response, survival, and safety with imatinib mesylate therapy in chronic-phase chronic myeloid leukemia after failure of interferon-α treatment. *Blood,* 111:1039-1043.

[21] Breccia M, Stefanizzi C, Cannella L, Latagliata R, Frustaci AM, Carmosino I, Santopiertro M, Alimena G (2008). Differences in hematological and non-hematological toxicity during treatment with imatinib in patients with early and late chronic phase chronic myeloid leukemia. *Leukemia & Lymphoma,* 49:2328-2332.

[22] Petzer AL, Wolf D, Fong D, Lion T, Dyagil I, masliak Z, Bogdanovic A, Griskevicius L, Lejniece S, Goranov S, Gercheva L, Stojanovic A, Peytchev D, Tzvetkov N, Griniute R, Oucheva R, Ulmer H, Kwakkelstein M, Rancati F, Gastl G (2010) High-dose imatinib improves cytogenetic and molecular remissions in patients with pretreated Philadelphia-positive, BCR-ABL-positive chronic phase chronic myeloid leukemia: first results from the randomized CELSG phase III CML 11 "ISTAHIT" study. *Haematologica*, 95:908-913.

[23] Palandri F, Castagnetti F, Testoni N, Luatti S, Marzocchi G, Bassi S, Breccia M, Alimena G, Pungolino E, Rege-Cambrin G, Varaldo R, Miglino M, Specchia G, Zuffa E, Ferrara F, Bocchia M, Saglio G, Pane F, Alberti D, Martinelli G, Baccarani M, Rosti G (2008). Chronic myeloid leukemia in blast crisis treated with imatinib 600 mg: outcome of the patients alive after a 6-year follow-up. *Haematologica,* 93: 1792-1796

[24] Hochhaus A, O'Brien SG, Guilhot F, Druker BJ, Branford S, Foroni L, Goldman JM, Muller MC, Radich JP, Rudolz M, Mone M, Gathmann I, Hughes TP, Larson RA (2009). Six-year follow-up of patients receiving imatinib for the first-line treatment of chronic myeloid leukemia. *Leukemia,* 23: 1054-1061.

[25] Hamdan MY, Sanders L, Olivera S, Campbell U, Willey V, Hirji I, Davis C, Ulcickas Yood M (2007). Discontinuation and dose modification of imatinib in clinical practice. J Clin Oncol, ASCO Annual Meeting Proceedings Part I. Vol 25, No. 18S (June 20 Supplement): 7045.

[26] Marin D, Marktel S, Bua M, Szydlo RM, Franceschino A, Nathan I, Foot N, Crawley C, Na Nakom T, Olavarria E, Lennard A, neylon A, O'Brien SH, Goldman JM, Apperley JF (2003) Prognostic factors for patients with chronic myeloid leukaemia in chronic phase treated with imatinib mesylate after failure of interferon alfa. *Leukemia,* 17:1448-1453.

[27] Sneed TB, Kantarjian HM, Talpaz M, O'Brien S, Rios MB, Bekele BN, Zhou X, Resta D, Wierda W, Faderl S, Giles F, Cortes JE (2003). The significance of myelosuppression during therapy with imatinib mesylate in patients with chronic myelogenous leukemia in chronic phase. *Cancer,* 100:116-121.

[28] Jabbour E, Deininger M, Hochhaus A (2011). Management of adverse events associated with tyrosine kinase inhibitors in the treatment of chronic myeloid leukemia. *Leukemia,* 25:201-210.

[29] Deininger MWN, O'Brien SG, Ford JM, Druker BJ (2003). Practical management of patients with chronic myeloid leukemia receiving imatinib. J Clin Oncol 24:1637-1647.
[30] NCCN Clinical Practice Guidelines in Oncology: Chronic Myelogenous Leukemia. V2.2011. Available from: http://www.nccn.org.
[31] Quintas-Cardama A, Kantarjian H, O'Brien S, Garcia-Manero G, Rios MB, Talpaz M, Cortes J (2004). Granulocyte-colonoy-stimulating factor (Filgrastim) may overcome imatinib-induced neutropenia in patients with chronic-phase chronic myelogenous leukemia. *Cancer,* 100:2592-2597.
[32] Marin D, Marktel S, Foot N, Bua M, Olavarria E, Goldman JM, Apperley JF (2003). Granulocyte colony-stimulating factor reverses cytopenia and may permit cytogenetic responses in patients with chronic myeloid leukemia treated with imatinib mesylate. *Haematologica,* 88:227-228.
[33] Jørgensen HG, Copland M, Holyoake TL (2005). Granulocyte-colony-stimulating factor (Filgrastim) may overcome imatinib-induced neutropenia in patients with chronic-phase myelogenous leukemia: letter to the editor. *Cancer,* 103:210-2011.
[34] Cortes j, O'Brien S, Quintas A, Giles F, Shan J, Rios MB, Talpaz M, Kantarjian H (2004). Erythropoietin is effective in improving the anemia induced by imatinib mesylate therapy in patients with chronic myeloid leukemia in chronic phase. *Cancer,* 100:2396-2402.
[35] Santos FPS, Alvarado Y, Kantarjian H, Verma D, O'Brien S, Mattiuzzi G, Ravandi F, Borthakur G, Cortes J (2011). Long-term prognostic impact of the use of erythropoietin-stimulating agents in patients with chronic myeloid leukemia in chronic phase treated with imatinib. *Cancer,* 117:982-991.
[36] Hassarjian RP, Boecklin F, Parker S, Chase A, Dhar S, Zaiac M, Olavarria E, Lampert I, Henry K, Apperley JF, Goldman JM (2002). STI571 (Imatinib mesylate) reduces bone marrow cellularity and normalizes morphologic features irrespective of cytogenetic response. *Hematopathology,* 117:360-367.
[37] Srinivas U, Pillai LS, Kumar R, Pati HP, Saxena R (2007). Bone marrow aplasia – A rare complication of imatinib therapy in CML patients. *Amer. J. Hem.,* 82:314-316.
[38] Chng WJ, Tan LHC (2005). Late-onset marrow aplasia due to imatinib in newly diagnosed chronic phase chronic myeloid leukaemia: Letter to the editor. *Leuk. Res.,* 29:719-720.
[39] Lokeshwar N, Kumar L, Kumari M (2005). Severe bone marrow aplasia following imatinib mesylate in a patient with chronic myelogenous leukemia. *Leukemia & Lymphoma,* 46:781-784.
[40] Ram R, Gafter-Gvili A, Okon E, pazgal I, Shpilberg O, Raanani P (2008). Gelatinous transformation of bone marrow in chronic myeloid leukemia during treatment with imatinib mesylate: A disease or a drug effect? *Acta. Haematol.,* 119:104-107
[41] Thakral B, Higa B, Venkataraman G, Velankar MM (2012). Bone marrow with gelatinous transformation associated with residual disease in imatinib mesylate-trated chronic myelogenous leukaemia (CML). Pathology 44:59.
[42] Tamura T, Tasaka T, Fujimoto M, Matshuhashi Y, Fukumot T, Mano S, Kuwajima M, Nagar M (2004). Massive bone marrow necrosis in a patient with chronic myelocytic leukemia following imatinib mesylate therapy. *Haematologica,* 89:109-110.

[43] Mastue K, Takeuchi M, Koseki M, Uryu H 2006. Bone marrow necrosis associated with the use of imatinib mesylate in a patient with Philadelphia chromosome-positive acute lymphoblastic leukemia: Letter to the Editor. *Ann. Hematol.,* 85:542-544.

[44] Vesterby A, Myhre Jensen O (1985). Asceptic bone/bone marrow necrosis in leukaemia. *Scand. J. Haematol.,* 35:354-357.

[45] Chim CS, Ma SK, Lam CK (1999). Bone marrow necrosis masquerading as interferon toxicity in chronic myeloid leukemia. *Leuk. Lymphoma,* 33:385-388

[46] Aras Y, Akcakaya MO, Unal SN, Bilgic B, Unal OF (2012). Bone marrow necrosis secondary to imatinib usage, mimicking spinal metastasis on magnetic resonance imaging and FDG-PET/CT. J. *Neurosurg.,:* Spine 16:57-60.

[47] Vanel D, Bonvalot S, Le Pechoux C, Cioffi A, Domont J, Le Cesne A (2007) Imatinib-induced bone marrow necrosis detected on MRI examination and mimicking bone metastasis. *Skeletal. Radiol.,* 36:895-898.

[48] De Arriba JJ, Nerin C, Garcia E, Gomez-Aldaravi L, Vila B (2003). Severe hemolytic anemia and skin reaction in a patient treated with imatinib. Annals of Oncology 14:962

[49] Zago Novaretti MC, Fonseca GHH, Conchon M, Dorlhiac-Llacer PE, de Alencar Fischer Chamone D (2003). First case of immune-mediated haemolytic anaemia associated to imatinib mesylate. *Haematology,* 71:455-458.

[50] Al Aly Z, Philoctete Ashley JM, Gellens ME, Gonzalez EA (2005). Thrombotic thrombocytopenic purpura in a patient treated with imatinib mesylate: true association or mere coincidence? *Am. J. Kidney Dis.,* 45:762-768.

[51] Schallier D, Trullemans F, Fontaine C, Decoster L, De Greve J (2009). Tyrosine kinase inhibitor-induced macrocytosis. *Anticancer Research,* 29:5225-5228.

[52] Aliberti S, Grignani G, Allione P, Vormola R, Bucci A, Porrino G, Ricchiardi A, Carnevale Schianca F, Rota Scalabrini D, Aglietta M (2005). Erythrocyte macrocytosis is a rather common, apparently uneventful yet unexplained finding in GIST imatinib (I) chronic therapy. J Clin Oncol, *ASCO Annual Meeting Proceedings*, 23(16S):9045.

[53] Hamberg P, Dulfer R, Oosten A, von Lindern MM, boere IA, van Doorn L, Meerten EV, Sleijfer S, Verweij J, Kruit WH (2010). Predictive and mechanistic factors of tyrosine kinase inhibitor (TKI) – induced macrocytosis. *J. Clin. Oncol.,* ASCO Annual Meeting Proceedings (Post-Meeting Edition) 28(15S):3052.

In: Imatinib
Editors: Mojtaba Akhtari and Ihab Elhemaidi
ISBN: 978-1-62808-297-5

Chapter 5

Cutaneous Adverse Events Related to Treatment with Imatinib

Paola Savoia*[*] *and Paolo Fava
Department of Biomedical Sciences and Human Oncology, Section of Dermatology, University of Turin, Torino, Italia

Abstract

Imatinib mesylate, (formally known as STI-571) is a 2-phenylaminopyrimidine derivative that operates as a selective inhibitor of PDGF-beta and Bcr-Abl oncogene; it is commonly used in the treatment of chronic myelogenous leukemia (CML), gastrointestinal stromal tumours (GIST), gliomas, small cell cancer and in unresecable or relapsed dermatofibrosarcoma protuberans (DFSP). Treatment with imatinib is generally well-tolerated, and in the majority of patients side effects are only represented by mild to moderate hematological toxicity. Edema is also a common drug related reaction reported in literature. Moreover, a wide spectrum of cutaneous reactions related to Imatinib administration has been recently described, including dose-dependent rash, pruritus, exfoliative dermatitis and edema. Hyperpigmentation of the skin and of the hair have been reported, as well as a localized repigmentation of areas involved by vitiligo. Localized or diffuse hypopigmentation was noted especially in ethnically pigmented CML patients and started after 2-12 weeks from the initiation of therapy. In Caucasian patients, an increased photosensibility was reported, but only a few cases of vitiligo-like lesions onset are described, together with uncommon cases of Halo Nevi. Imatinib-related skin depigmentation could be explained in at least two different ways: STI-571 can inhibit c-kit tyrosine kinase functions in melanocytes in vitro; Imatinib can also reduce indirectly melanocytes proliferation, decreasing the secretion of melanogenic molecules by skin fibroblasts. However, the pathogenesis of cutaneous disorders related to treatment with imatinib is not fully explained and the immune system activation status could play a central role. In this chapter, a thorough description of cutaneous adverse events related to Imatinib treatment will be provided and the more intriguing pathogenesis hypotheses will be extensively discussed.

[*] Corresponding author: Tel. 011/6335816, Fax 011/6335034, Email: paola.savoia@unito.it.

Introduction

Treatment with Imatinib is generally well-tolerated, and in the majority of patients side effects are only represented by mild to moderate hematological toxicity (Druker 2001).

However, a wide spectrum of cutaneous reaction related to imatinib administration has been reported in recent literature. In this chapter, a thorough description of cutaneous adverse events related to Imatinib treatment is provided and the pathogenetics hypothesis will be discussed.

Incidence

Cutaneous adverse effects from Imatinib are relatively common, but the incidence reported by the literature studies is various. The rate of cutaneous adverse effects reported from Druker (2001) is of 17% for rash and 39% for edema, whereas Van Oosterom (2001) and Valerye (2003) report an incidence of 55% and 65% respectively. These differences might be explained by the different doses of Imatinib used in the various trials: in fact, the incidence of cutaneous reactions to Imatinib appears to be dose-dependent, suggesting that they are related to the pharmacologic effect of the drug rather than to hypersensitivity phenomena (Brourad 2001). The prevalence of cutaneous side effects was significantly higher in females, as generally reported also for other skin drug reactions.

Cutaneous Adverse Effects

Cutaneous adverse effects represent 7-21% of all toxic events (Brourad 2001). The majority of skin reactions are grade mild to moderate and only in 5% of cases they are life-threatening.

Pruritus is not dose-dependent and occurs in more than 40% of patients treated with Imatinib as an isolated finding or in association to other cutaneous manifestations; however, in the majority of patients, pruritus is mild to moderate and only in few cases treatment was withdrawn due to the severity of reaction (Valerye 2003).

Dose-dependent skin rash is the most commonly described side-effect, and usually occurs within the first 12 weeks of treatment (Breccia 2005). The majority of patients develop a grade II dermatitis, with erythema associated to desquamation and moderate edema; grade III or IV reaction, with confluent erythematous-desquamative lesions are relatively rare. Cutaneous dryness and cheilitis affect a fair number of patients.

Edema is a common drug-related reaction that occurs in a percentage of patients varying from 48% to 65% (Valerye 2003; Arora 2004), after a time of approximately 6 weeks from the beginning of treatment. In the majority of cases, edema is localized to peri-ocular region or on the lower limb, but also cases of generalized edema are described. Only in a small percentage of patient edema is associated with severe liquid retention, even if a weight increase is described in 26% of patients without clinically evident edema. Edema is significantly related to daily dose, whereas no relationship with sex, age or weight at the beginning of the treatment has been observed (Valerye 2003).

Even if skin rash and edema are the most frequently cutaneous adverse events reported, a number of rare cutaneous reactions related to Imatinib have been described.

Pseudoporphyria is a rare bullous disease with clinical, histological and immunofluorecence features mimicking *Porphyria cutanea tarda* in absence of alterations in porphyrin metabolism. Usually pseudoporphyria is associated to the use of medications such as naproxen or other non-steroideal anti-inflammatory drugs, but a case of Imatinib induced pseudoporphyria was recently described (Timmer-de Mik 2008) in a 42-year-old male affected by chronic myeloid leukaemia (CML). Moreover, a erythematous eruption on the photoexposed areas, with clinical and histopatological features of drug-photoinducted dermatitis, was described after 1 year of treatment with Imatinib in a patients affected by CLM, who developed also an unusual oral lichenoid reaction (Brazzelli 2012). The molecular mechanism of the Imatinib induced photosensitivity will be analyzed further.

Another recent paper reports three cases of Imatinib related pytiriasis rosea-like eruption in CML patients, characterized by a erythematous slightly pruritic, macular skin eruption confined to trunk, limbs and arms (Brazzelli 2005). In literature, drug related cutaneous lesions resembling pytiriasis rosea have been previously described as a consequence of methoxypromazina, barbiturate, clonidine, captopril, omeprazole, isotretinoine, D-penicillamine and terbinafine.

Moreover, a patient with a metastatic gastro-intestinal stromal tumor (GIST) developed painful erythemato-edematous lesions located on soles and palms three weeks after Imatinib treatment initiation and followed by onychomadesis of all the nails. The eruption promptly resolved with topical clobetasol propionate without Imatinib discontinuation (Battistella 2008). A case of Imatinib related acute generalized exanthematous pustolosis (AGEP) is also described; this is a drug reaction characterized by a febrile disseminated macular eruption with aseptic non-follicular pustules mainly located on the trunk (Brouard 2001).

Some painful mucosal erosions associated to lichenoid reactions have also been described (Lim 2002, Pascual 2006, Basso 2008), such as three cases of livedoid skin reactions (Martinez-Gonzalez 2007).

Valerye et al. describe 4 cases of Imatinib-induced psoriasis; only 2 of these patients had a previous history of psoriasis. Deguchi et al reported other three cases of psoriasiform palmoplantar hyperkeratosis with nail distrophy in CML patients without previous history of psoriasis. Actually, the effects of Imatinb on psoriasis need to be clarified: Miyagawa et.al (33 reviews) reports instead a case of Imatinib-induced improvement in psoriatic patients affected by GIST.

Severe reactions that are reported include Steven-Johonson syndrome, GVHD-like syndrome and SCC carcinoma (Hsiao 2002, Schaich 2003, Baskaynak 2003), but fortunately they are rare.

Generally, the majority of skin reactions are self-limiting or easily managed with a low dose corticosteroid regimen (oral prednisone 10-20 mg daily). In a few patients with grade IV dermatosis, in which high doses (50 mg daily) of prednisone were unsuccessfully administrated, a suspension or a definitive interruption of Imatinib could be required.

Usually, edema could be easily managed by limiting salt intake or by diuretics; an improvement of peri-ocular edema with topical phenylephrine 0.25% is also described.

Pigmentary Disorders

Pigmentary disorders are reported in about 40% of patients during Imatinib treatment (Arora 2004), within a median time of 4 weeks from the therapy initiation.

Treatment related hypo- and hyper-pigmentation are described mainly in ethnically pigmented patients. Hasan et al. reported the case of a black Nigerian male affected by GIST who developed depigmentation on the fingertips and Tsao et al described a loss of pigmentation in other six Afro Americans patients affected by CML. The pigmentation changes develop within one month from the start of treatment and persist during therapy; from a clinical point of view, hypopigmentation can be generalized or located in patches on the face, arms or trunk imatinib mesilate-induced hypopigmentation is dose-related and reversible: dose reduction leaded to darkening of skin pigmentation. Interestingly, in one of these CML patients, hypopigmentation regressed when treatment was interrupted, but occurred again at the imatinib restart.

In Caucasian patients pigmentary disorders are reported more rarely. Raanani et al (Raanani 2002) described the hypopigmentation of the distal part of both hands and the penis in a chronic myeloid leukaemia patient and Brazzelli et al vitiligo-like lesions occurred in a 17-year-old Caucasian patient after 5 months Imatinib treatment. A generalized loss of pigmentation was also described after 6 months of treatment with Imatinib in a 46-year- old Caucasian women with chronic myeloid leukemia (Brazzelli 2007).

Our group previously described a 46-year-old Caucasian male patient successfully treated with imatinib for a dermatofibrosarcoma (DFSP) who developed depigmentation areas around some nevi. This phenomenon, that represent the clinical result of a lymphohistiocytic inflammatory infiltrate against melanocytes and arise more frequently in children and young adults, was initially limited to the back, but in a few weeks halo nevi developed diffusely, with histological documented signs of regression, associated with infiltration by lymphocytes, macrophages and neutrophils. Imatinib was discontinued after 9 months of treatment, when tumour became surgically treatable; despite the prompt resolution of periorbital edema, halo nevi persisted from more than 3 months from suspension (Fava 2010). Hair depigmentation has also been reported (Huang 2009).

Hyperpigmentation of the skin is rare, affecting about 3% of Imatinib-treated CML patients from the series described by Arora at al. This pigmentation can be diffused and histologically is characterized by the presence of dermal melanophages; a localized darkening of hair color was also described (Etienne 2000, Valerye 2003), as well as a spotted repigmentation of areas involved by vitiligo (Han 2008).

Recently, a case in which patches with clinical features suggesting acne rosacea developed together with diffuse hyperpigmentation of the face was also reported (Demirci 2010)

Pathogenesis

The mechanisms of skin toxicity from imatinib are complex and still debated. Many hypotheses have been proposed in order to explain the different molecular pathways involved in the onset of these reactions.

In regard to the effects of imatinib on the pathogenesis of psoriasis and the other inflammatory cutaneous reactions, further studies are needed. However, it is well known that T lymphocytes play a crucial role both in psoriasis and inflammatory dermatoses. There is also evidence of the pathogenetic involvement of PDGF and Stem Cell Factor (SCF) in the disease (Dickens 2009). Cytokine production and T cell proliferation are affected by imatinib. The drug inhibits interferon-c secretion by T effector cells, but the function of these cells is modulated rather than suppressed (Valerye 2003). These effects, together with imatinib's suppression of c-Kit and PDGFR, may help to explain the exacerbation of psoriasis in some patients.

Regarding the pathogenesis of Imatinib-related cutaneous side effects, it has been suggested that they could be mediated by a pharmacological effect. Indeed, the drug acts directly on the PDGF receptor expressed on blood vessels negatively regulating transcapillary transport. Moreover, an Imatinib-mediated inhibition of this receptor may cause an increase of dermal interstitial fluid pressure, with the onset of edema and subsequently, erythema and desquamation (Pietras 2001).

Imatinib can have an affect on skin pigmentation in different and more subtle ways. The drug can inhibit c-Kit tyrosinase kinase function in melanocytes or reduce indirectly the melanocytes proliferation decreasing melanogenic molecules secretion by cutaneous fibroblasts (Cario-André 2003). C-Kit is routinely expressed in normal melanocytes, in benign nevi, dysplastic nevi and melanoma; on the contrary in epidermidis affected by the vitiligo Kit, expression results were reduced. Moreover, a constitutive signaling from the c-Kit receptor did not stimulate melanogenesis and proliferation, but significantly promoted migration of the melanocytes both in vitro and in vivo; thus, activation of the c-Kit receptor tyrosine kinase may antagonize proliferation and melanogenesis (Alexeev 2006). The activation of Kit initiates a signaling cascade that results in the phosphorylation of the Microphthalmia-associated transcription factor (Mitf) and a concomitant increase in its transcriptional activation activity (Goding 2000). These mechanisms can be implicated in Imatinib-related skin depigmentation, even if they don't completely explain the onset of vitiligo or halo nevi in these patients.

References

Alexeev, V; Yoon, K. Distinctive role of the cKit receptor tyrosine kinase signaling in mammalian melanocytes. *J Invest Dermatol.* 2006; 126, 945-947.

Arora, B; Kumar, L; Sharma, A; Wadhwa, J; Kochupillai, V. Pigmentary changes in chronic myeloid leukemia patients treated with imatinib mesylate. *Ann Oncol.* 2004; 15, 358-359.

Baskaynak, G; Kreuzer, KA; Schwarz, M; et al. Squamous cutaneous epithelial cell carcinoma in two CML patients with progressive disease under imatinib treatment. *Eur J Haematol*, 2003; 70, 231–234.

Basso, FG; Boer, CC; Corrêa, ME; Torrezan, M; et al. Skin and oral lesions associated to imatinib mesylate therapy. *Support Care Cancer.* 2009, 17, 465-468.

Battistella, M; Frémont, G; Vignon-Pennamen, MD; Gornet, JM; Dubertret, L; Viguier, M. Imatinib-Induced Hand-Foot Syndrome in a Patient With Metastatic Gastrointestinal Stromal Tumor. *Arch Dermatol.* 2008; 144, 1400-1402.

Brazzelli, V; Prestinari, F; Roveda, E; et al. Pityriasis rosea-like eruption during treatment with imatinib mesylate: description of 3 cases. *J Am Acad Dermatol*, 2005; 53, S240–S243.

Brazzelli, V; Roveda, E; Prestinari, F; et al. Vitiligo-like lesions and diffuse lightening of the skin in a pediatric patien treated with Imatinib mesylate: a non-invasive colorimetric assessment. *Ped Dermatol*, 2006; 23, 175-178.

Brazzelli, V; Prestinari, F; Barbagallo, T; et al. A long-term time course of colorimetric assessment of the effects of imatinib mesylate on skin pigmentation: a study of five patients. *J Eur Acad Dermatol Venereol*, 2007; 21, 384–387.

Brazzelli, V; Muzio1, F; Manna1, G; et al. Photoinduced dermatitis and oral lichenoid reaction in a chronic myeloid leukemia patient treated with imatinib mesylate. *Photodermatology, Photoimmunology & Photomedicine*, 2012; 28, 2–5.

Breccia, M; Latagliata, R; Carmosino, I; Mandelli, F; Alimena, G. Reactivation of porphyria cutanea tarda as a possible side effect of Imatinib at high dosage in chronic myeloid leukemia. *Leukemia*. 2004; 18, 182.

Brourad, M; Saurat, JH. Cutaneous reactions to STI571. *N Engl J Med*, 2001; 345, 618-619.

Cario-Andrě, M; Pain, C; Gauthier, Y; et al. In vivo and in vitro evidence of dermal fibroblasts influence on human epidermal pigmentation. *Pigment Cell Res*, 2006; 19, 434-442.

Demirci, U; Coskun, U; Erdem, O; et al. Acne rosacea associated imatinib mesylate in a gastrointestinal stromal tumor patient. *J Oncol Pharm Pract*. 2011; 17, 285-287.

Dickens, E; Lewis, F; Bienz, N. Imatinib: a designer drug, another cutaneous complication. *Clin Exp Dermatol*. 2009; 34, 603-604.

Druker, BJ; Talpaz, M; Resta, DJ; et al. Efficacy and safety of a specific inhibitor of the BCR-ABL tyrosine kinase in chronic myeloid leukemia. *N Engl J Med*, 2001; 344, 1031-1037.

Etienne, G; Cony-Makhoul, P; Mahon, FX. Imatinib mesylate and gray hair. *N Engl J Med*. 2002, 8; 347, 446.

Fava, P; Stroppiana, E; Savoia, P; Bernengo, MG. Halo nevi related to treatment with imatinib in a dermatofibrosarcoma protuberans patient. *J Eur Acad Dermatol Venereol*. 2010; 24, 244-245.

Goding, CR. Mitf from neural crest to melanoma: signal transduction and transcription in the melanocyte lineage. *Genes Dev*. 2000 Jul 15; 14(14), 1712-1728.

Gonçalves Basso, F; Cominato Boer, C; et al. Skin and oral lesions associated to imatinib mesylate therapy. *Support care cancer*, 2008; doi 10.1007/s00520-008-0536-8.

Han, H; Yu, YY; Wang, Y. Imatinib mesylate-induced repigmentation of vitiligo lesions in a patient with recurrent gastrointestinal stromal tumors. *J Am Acad Dermatol*, 2008; 59, 80-83.

Hasan, S; Dinh, K; Lombardo, F; et al. Hypopigmentation in an African patient treated with imatinib mesylate: a case report. *J Natl Med Assoc*, 2003; 95, 722–724.

Hsiao, LT; Chung, HM; Lin, JT; et al. Stevens-Johnson syndrome after treatment with STI571: a case report. *Br J Haematol*, 2002; 117, 620–622.

Huang, X; Patel, S; Ahmed, N; Seiter, K; Liu, D. Severe toxicity of skin rash, fever and diarrhea associated with imatinib: case report and review of skin toxicities associated with tyrosine kinase inhibitors. *Drug Des Devel Ther*. 2009, 6; 2, 215-219.

Lim, DS; Muir, J. Oral lichenoid reaction to imatinib (STI 571, Gleevec). *Dermatology*, 2002; 205, 169–171.

Martínez-González, MC; del Pozo, J; Yebra-Pimentel, MT; Pérez, M; Almagro, M; Fonseca, E. Livedoid Skin Reaction Probably Due to Imatinib Therapy. *Ann Pharmacother*, 2007; 41, 148-152.

Pascual, JC; Matarredona, J; Miralles, J; et al. Oral and cutaneous lichenoid reaction secondary to imatinib: report of two cases. *Int J Dermatol*, 2006; 45, 1471–1473.

Pietras, K; Ostman, A; Sjoquist, M; et al. Inhibition of platelet derived growth factor receptors reduces interstitial hypertension and increases transcapillary transport in tumors. *Cancer Res*, 2001; 61, 2929–2934.

Raanani, P; Goldman, JM; Ben.Bassat, I. Challanges in oncology. Case 3. Depigmentation in a chronic myeloid leukaemia patient treated with STI-571. *J Clin Oncol*. 2002; 20, 869-870.

Schaich, M; Schakel, K; Illmer, T; Ehninger, G; Bornhauser, M. Severe epidermal necrolysis after treatment with imatinib and consecutive allogeneic hematopoietic stem cell transplantation. *Ann Hematol*, 2003; 82, 303–304.

Timmer-de Mik, L; Kardaun, SH; Kramer, MHH; Hayes, DP; Bousema, MT. Imatinib-induced pseudoporphyria. *Clin Exp Dermatol*, 2008; 1-3.

Tsao, AS; Kantarjian, H; Cortes, J; et al. Imatinib mesylate causes hypopigmentation in the skin. *Cancer*, 2003; 98, 2483–2487.

Valeyrie, L; Bastuji-Garin, S; Revuz, J; et al. Adverse cutaneous reactions to imatinib (STI571) in Philadelphia chromosome-positive leukemias: a prospective study of 54 patients. *J Am Acad Dermatol*. 2003; 48, 201-206.

Van Oosterom; Judson, I; Verweij, J; et al. Safety and efficacy of imatinib (STI571) in metastatic gastrointestinal stromal cancers: a phase I study. *Lancet*, 2001; 358, 1421-1423.

In: Imatinib
Editors: Mojtaba Akhtari and Ihab Elhemaidi
ISBN: 978-1-62808-297-5

Chapter 6

The Skeletal Effects of Imatinib Mesylate

Susannah O'Sullivan* and Andrew Grey
Department of Medicine, University of Auckland, Auckland, New Zealand

Abstract

Imatinib mesylate (Glivec^{TM}), and the related tyrosine kinase inhibitors (TKIs) nilotinib and dasatinib, are now standard care for the treatment Chronic Myeloid Leukemia (CML) and it is likely that most patients will remain on one of these agents indefinitely. In addition imatinib is utilised in the treatment of gastrointestinal stromal cells tumor (GIST) and disorders that are characterized by activated PDGF receptor signalling. "Bystander effects" due to inhibition of imatinib's target receptors in normal tissues have been observed, including effects on bone and calcium metabolism. *In vitro*, imatinib has effects on osteoblast proliferation, survival and differentiation, and osteoclastogenesis, through inhibition of the PDGFR and c-fms. Some data from animal studies demonstrate reduced bone formation and bone mass after treatment with imatinib. Humans treated with imatinib develop secondary hyperparathyroidism and reduced levels of markers of bone turnover. In adult humans imatinib has a neutral or positive effect on bone mass, and data are largely reassuring regarding the safety of medium-term use for treatment of CML or GIST. In children, there may be negative effects of imatinib on growth. Here we review the skeletal effects of imatinib and discuss the possible mechanisms for these effects. Given the potential for patients to receive imatinib in the long term, we consider the implications of these effects for bone health in such patients.

Introduction

Imatinib mesylate (Glivec^{TM}), formerly referred to as STI571, is an orally active tyrosine kinase inhibitor (TKI) that has revolutionized drug therapy of chronic myeloid leukemia

* Email: s.osullivan@auckland.ac.nz; Ph: 64-9-9236138, Fax: 64-9-3737677.

(CML), having been shown to be an effective treatment for all stages of the disease [1-6]. Imatinib has positive long-term effects on progression-free and overall survival compared to other treatments [7-9], although efficacy is compromised in some patients by the development of resistance [10-12] and/or adverse effects leading to poor adherence [13, 14]. 20-25% of newly diagnosed patients do not reach complete cytogenetic remission implying disease resistance [15] and a further 20–25% of those who do achieve complete hematological response and/or complete cytogenetic remission will acquire resistance to imatinib [12]. Both these outcomes are more likely in patients treated with imatinib for the first time in the accelerated or blastic phases [12]. Approximately one third of patients have been found to be non-adherent [14, 16]. *BCR-ABL* positive cells are detectable in more than 95% of patients treated with imatinib who achieve complete cytogenetic remission [17]. These cells are resistant to imatinib and potentially provide a source of future disease progression. Discontinuation of imatinib is associated with moderate relapse rates [18], thus many patients will receive the drug indefinitely.

In addition to activity against all abl tyrosine kinases (TKs) [19-21], imatinib inhibits the platelet-derived growth factor (PDGF) receptors α and β [19, 22], c-kit [19, 23] and c-fms at therapeutic concentrations [24, 25]. Hence, it has an established role in the treatment of gastrointestinal stromal cells tumor (GIST) [26-29], and several disorders that are characterized by activated PDGF receptor signalling [30-32], and is being investigated as a treatment for other metabolic, inflammatory and proliferative conditions [33-38]. "Bystander effects" have been observed in animals and humans receiving imatinib, due to inhibition of imatinib's target receptors in normal tissues. The most common of these are hypopigmentation and diarrhoea, and male hypogonadism has also been reported, all due to inhibition of c-kit [15, 39-41]. Hematologic side effects have been observed in CML patients treated with imatinib [15], and there has been a report of cardiotoxicity attributed to inhibition of c-abl [42]. Other bystander effects include fluid retention, hypoglycaemia, and liver toxicity [15, 43, 44].

Indirect evidence suggested that imatinib might affect bone and mineral metabolism. In male patients treated with imatinib for CML, the low testosterone levels that have been observed [39], have the potential to lead to bone loss. Imatinib's target TKs are present in bone and play roles in normal bone metabolism. c-abl is a widely expressed protein, with high levels being found in hyaline cartilage in the adult, bone tissue in newborn mice, and osteoblasts in the fetus [45, 46]. Li et al have demonstrated that $Abl^{-/-}$ mice are osteoporotic as a result of decreased bone formation due to impaired osteoblast differentiation [47]. PDGF is regarded as an important osteogenic factor, involved in the recruitment of osteoprogenitor cells, and their proliferation and differentiation into mature osteoblasts [48-50]. The PDGF-BB isomer has a growth-promoting effect on osteoclasts, associated with an increase in bone eroded surface [51, 52]. PDGF's role in bone *in vivo* is not well characterised due to embryonic lethality in many transgenic models [53-56]. When PDGF is administered to wild-type animals, it has been found to increase bone formation and accelerate fracture healing [57, 58]. Stem cell factor (SCF) the ligand for c-kit, has been shown to increase the proliferation of osteoclast precursors, suggesting that it may play a role in enhancing/expanding the precursor pool [59-61], and to stimulate osteoclastic bone resorption [59, 60]. A study of SCF mutant mice (Sl/Sl^d), which lack the membrane-bound form of SCF, reported an osteopenic phenotype, attributed to a reduction in osteoblast proliferation and, to a lesser extent, differentiation, and a decrease in osteoblast activity. In contrast, there was an increase in late stage osteoclast precursors [62]. Macrophage colony-stimulating factor (M-CSF) is one of the cytokines that is essential for osteoclastogenesis, contributing to precursor cell proliferation, survival and differentiation [63, 64]. The importance of M-CSF, the ligand of c-fms, in bone metabolism has been elaborated by analysis of the *op/op* mouse, which has a total absence of biologically active M-CSF, and is osteopetrotic due to an absence of osteoclasts and bone resorption [65].

Studies published by our group and others suggest that imatinib has important effects on bone and calcium metabolism [66-85]. *In vitro*, imatinib decreases osteoblast proliferation and survival, and increases osteoblast differentiation, actions which may be attributable to inhibition of PDGFR signaling [71-74, 79]. Imatinib decreases osteoclastogenesis *in vitro*, by both direct and indirect, stromal-cell dependent mechanisms [69, 72, 83, 85]. *In vivo* imatinib reduces bone formation and bone mass [75]. Studies of humans treated with imatinib show altered bone and mineral metabolism [76-82, 86] and a biphasic effect on bone turnover [76-78, 80, 81]. Four small studies of the effects of imatinib on bone mass in humans with CML suggest that imatinib has a neutral or possibly beneficial effect on the skeleton [76, 78, 79, 82]. Here we review the skeletal effects of imatinib and discuss the possible mechanisms for these effects. Given the potential for patients to receive imatinib in the long term, we consider the implications of these effects for bone health in such patients.

Effects of Imatinib on Osteoblasts

The cells that mediate bone formation are the osteoprogenitor cells (maintain the osteoblast population and bone mass), osteoblasts (synthesis of bone matrix), osteocytes (support bone structure and regulate osteoblast differentiation) and protective bone surface lining cells [87]. Bone formation involves osteoblast proliferation, differentiation and maturation. The growth of osteoblast progenitors, their differentiation to form mature osteoblasts and osteoblast activity and apoptosis are controlled by a number of factors, including steroid and polypeptide hormones, growth factors and cytokines.

Imatinib has potent anti-proliferative effects on osteoblastic and osteoprogenitor cells [71-74, 79]. Thus, at concentrations achieved *in vivo* with therapeutic doses of imatinib (0.01-1.0μM), there is a dose-dependent inhibition of proliferation in primary rat osteoblasts, stromal ST2 cells, and pre-osteoblastic MC3T3E1 cells [72] (Figures 1A and B). Similar effects are seen in human bone marrow mesenchymal stem cells (hBM-MSCs) and human bone explant cultures [71, 73, 74, 79].

At higher concentrations (1 - 5μM), imatinib promotes apoptosis of primary rat osteoblasts [72] (Figure 1C) although this effect was not seen in human bone explant cultures [79]. In contrast, imatinib stimulates differentiation and differentiated activity of osteoblasts [71-74, 79]. At similar doses to those that inhibit proliferation, imatinib dose-dependently increases differentiation of primary rat osteoblasts and MC3T3E1 cells, with a concurrent increase in mineralisation [72] (Figure 2A). In hBM-MSCs treated with therapeutically-achievable doses of imatinib there is an increase in osteoblast differentiation and mineralisation [73], while at higher doses there is inhibition of these processes [71, 74] An increase in mineral formation has been observed in human bone explant cultures treated with imatinib [79]. In keeping with these findings, quantitative analysis of the expression of genes known to reflect osteoblast differentiation confirms that at clinically-relevant doses imatinib accelerates and amplifies this process [72].

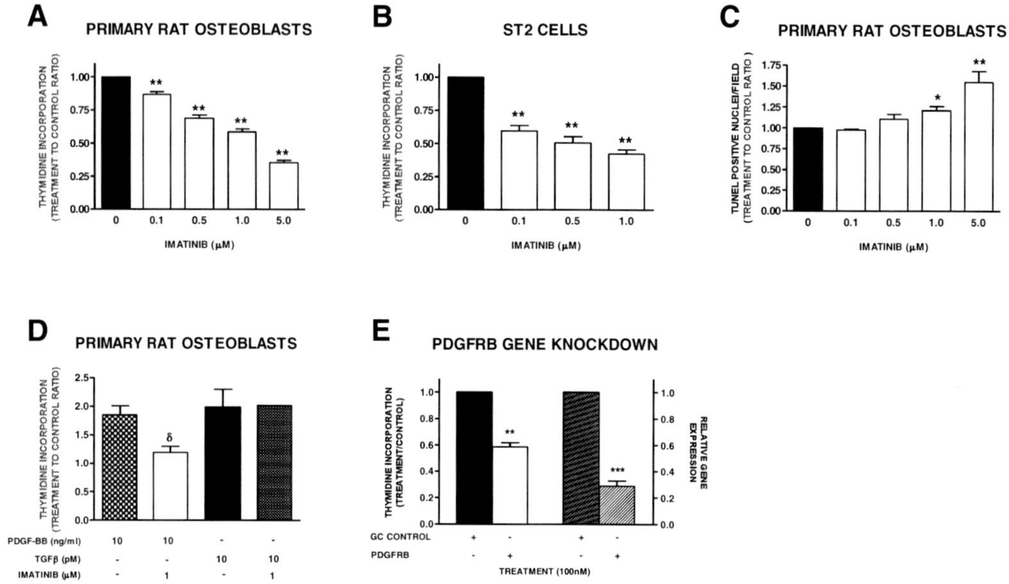

Figure 1. Effects of imatinib on [^{3}H]-thymidine incorporation in A) primary rat osteoblasts and B) ST2 stromal cells. Cells were cultured in 1% FCS during the 24 hour treatment with imatinib. Data are mean ± SEM. *, p<0.05 vs control; **, p<0.01 vs control. C) Effects of imatinib on apoptosis induced by serum deprivation in primary rat osteoblasts, as assessed by TUNEL. Data are mean ± SEM number of apoptotic nuclei per microscopic field. *, p<0.05 vs control. D) PDGF stimulates osteoblast proliferation, an effect inhibited by imatinib. Imatinib does not inhibit osteoblast proliferation induced by TGF-β. Data are mean ± SEM. **, p<0.01 vs control; δ, p<0.01 vs PDGF. E) Effects of siRNA targeting PDGFRB on [^{3}H]-thymidine incorporation in ST2 cells. Cells are treated with siRNA for PDGFRB or GC control sequence. Bars on left show [^{3}H]-thymidine incorporation, bars on right show gene expression, determined by q-PCR. Data are mean ± SEM. **, p<0.01 vs control oligo; ***, p<0.001 vs control oligo [72]. Reproduced with permission of American Society for Bone and Mineral Research.

Thus, expression of alkaline phosphatase (ALP), osteocalcin (OCN), and bone sialoprotein (BSP) were all increased by imatinib in primary rat osteoblasts cultured in mineralising conditions (Figure 2B). In human bone explant cultures, addition of imatinib significantly increased expression of the osteoblastogenic genes osteoblast specific transcription factor (osterix, OSX) and bone morphogenic protein 2 (BMP-2) [79]. In hBM-MSCs the levels of OCN, runt-related transcription factor 2 (Runx2/Cbfa1) and BMP-2 expression were increased in cells treated with imatinib [73], although there was a decrease at later time points in the osteoblastic genes Runx2 and Type I collagen when cells were treated with a higher dose of imatinib (5μM) [74].

It has been proposed that the mechanism of these osteoblastic effects of imatinib is via inhibition of the PDGFR-β. Recombinant PDGF enhances proliferation of primary rat osteoblasts, stromal ST2 cells, and pre-osteoblastic MC3T3E1 cells and increases thymidine incorporation in fetal rat calvarial organ cultures [72, 88, 89]. This effect is reversed by co-treatment with imatinib (Figure 1D) [72]. Of the other molecular targets, activation of c-kit by

SCF, has only a minimal stimulatory effect on proliferation in stromal ST2 cells and ABL-null osteoblasts proliferate normally [72, 90]. Furthermore, when PDGFRB gene and PDGFR-β protein expression is reduced using gene silencing techniques, there is a reduction in mitogenesis in ST2 cells (Figure 1E). This effect is not seen when there is a similar degree of inhibition of expression of genes encoding PDGFRA or ABL, and ST2 cells do not express the KIT gene [72, 90]. PDGFRβ-depletion in murine mesenchymal stem cells (MSC) led to decreased mitogenesis and enhanced osteogenic differentiation [91].

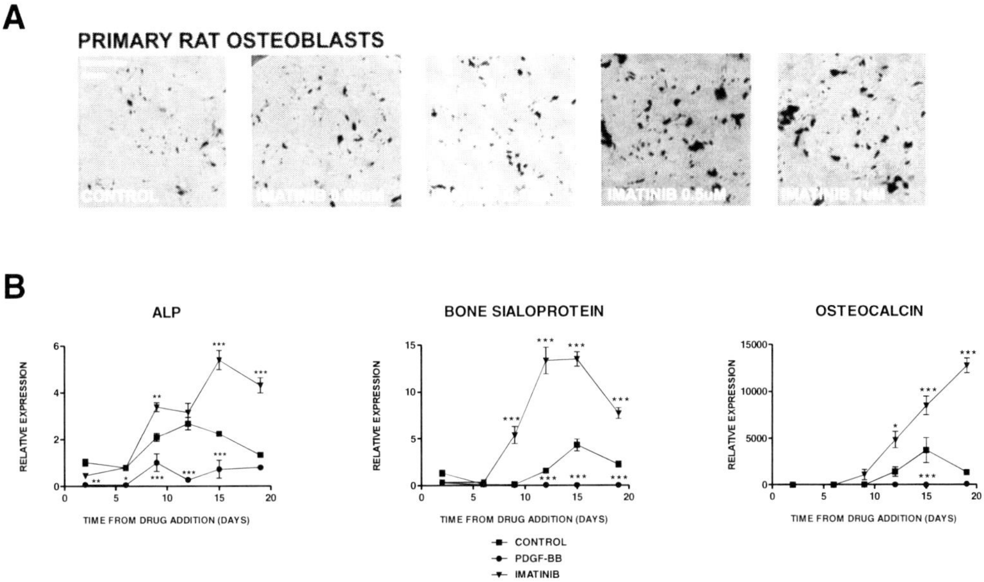

Figure 2. Effects of imatinib on A) differentiation of primary rat osteoblasts. Results of the differentiation assay are presented as micrographs showing mineralized nodules (black, von Kossa stain) in cultured osteoblastic cells. B) Effects of imatinib and PDGF-BB on expression of genes reflecting osteoblast differentiation in primary rat osteoblasts. Gene expression data are expressed relative to the day 2 control value. Data are mean ± SEM. *, $p<0.05$ vs control; **, $p<0.01$ vs control; ***, $p<0.001$ vs control [72]. Reproduced with permission of American Society for Bone and Mineral Research.

PDGF has also been shown to inhibit osteoblast differentiation. Thus PDGF-BB reduces mineralisation in MC3T3-E1 cells, hBM-MSC and primary rat osteoblasts [48, 72, 91, 92]. Furthermore it potently suppresses the expression of genes associated with osteoblast differentiation [72, 92] (Figure 2B). Co-treatment with imatinib completely reversed the inhibitory effects of PDGF on osteoblast differentiation [72]. By contrast, SCF has a mild stimulatory effect on osteoblast differentiation [72], and mice deficient in ABL have impaired osteoblast differentiation [47], suggesting that the PDGFR is the important imatinib target in mediating the stimulatory actions of the drug on osteoblast differentiation. Taken as a whole, these data suggest that PDGFR signalling in osteoblasts promotes expansion of the osteoblast precursor pool at the expense of osteoblast differentiation, and that imatinib therapy produces the opposite outcome.

Effects of Imatinib on Osteoclasts

Osteoclasts are giant multinucleated cells and are the sole bone resorptive cells. They originate from cells in the mononuclear/phagocytic lineage, the principal precursor being the bone marrow macrophage [93]. The ability of the mature osteoclast to resorb bone depends upon its ability to form a microenvironment between itself and the underlying bone matrix, and produce electrolytes and degradative enzymes essential to the resorptive process [93, 94]. Osteoclast precursor proliferation and maturation, and the function of mature osteoclasts can be influenced by local factors generated in the bone microenvironment, and by systemic hormones. Cytokines that are essential for osteoclastogenesis include receptor activator of nuclear factor kappa B ligand (RANKL) [95, 96] and M-CSF [97]. RANKL is a member of the tumour necrosis factor (TNF) family through which osteoblasts and marrow stromal cells interact with the receptor, receptor activator of nuclear factor kappa B (RANK), on marrow macrophages, driving them to assume the osteoclast phenotype. In addition it increases the osteoclast bone-resorbing activity of mature osteoclast and prolongs their survival [95, 98-100]. RANKL activity is negatively regulated by osteoprotegerin (OPG), a glycoprotein secreted by stromal cells which competes with RANK as a soluble decoy receptor [101]. The role of M-CSF is in assuring the proliferation and survival of macrophages [102]. M-CSF is required for commitment to the monocyte lineage, while stimulating proliferation of these precursors and expression of the RANK receptor [103].

Imatinib has consistently been shown to inhibit osteoclastogenesis *in vitro* [66-69, 72]. In murine bone marrow cultures, stimulated with $1,25(OH)_2D$, imatinib led to a reduction in the number of newly developed osteoclasts at concentrations of 0.1 μM and higher, and at 1 μM, imatinib completely abrogated osteoclastogenesis [72] (Figures 3A and B). A lesser effect was seen in stromal-cell independent cultures, such as murine bone marrow cultures incubated with recombinant M-CSF and RANK in the absence of $1,25(OH)_2D$, and cultures of the RAW-264.7 macrophage cell line [72] (Figure 3C). Imatinib also inhibits osteoclastogenesis in human CD14+ peripheral blood mononuclear cells and primary rat bone marrow cells at concentrations of 1 μM and greater [66, 69]. At higher doses (2.5 – 5μM) osteoclast survival is inhibited by imatinib [83]. Imatinib has also been shown to reduce the function of mature osteoclasts, as demonstrated by a reduction in their capacity to resorb a dentine substrate or bovine bone slice [69, 83].

A number of mechanisms have been proposed for imatinib's inhibition of osteoclast formation and function. A striking feature of the murine bone marrow cultures is a dose-dependent reduction in the number of stromal cells in the presence of imatinib, consistent with the anti-proliferative and pro-apoptotic effects that have been observed in pre-osteoblastic cells [72]. This finding suggests that imatinib may induce stromal cell-dependent inhibition of osteoclastogenesis by limiting the number of stromal cells available to support differentiation of osteoclast precursors. A further mechanism by which imatinib might indirectly inhibit osteoclastogenesis is by altering stromal cell production of cytokines known to influence osteoclast development [104]. OPG gene expression is significantly increased in cultures of primary rat osteoblasts treated with imatinib, and OPG protein secretion is increased in imatinib-treated ST2 cells (Figures 3D and E) [72]. The increase in OPG production by osteoblastic cells may also be the result of PDGFRβ inhibition. Treatment of ST2 cells with PDGF decreases OPG mRNA expression (Figure 3F), whereas silencing of the

PDGFRB gene in these same cells increases OPG mRNA expression (O'Sullivan, manuscript in preparation). These data suggest that an increase in OPG production by stromal/osteoblastic cells in response to imatinib may contribute to the anti-resorptive actions of the drug, and that this increase may be due to imatinib's inhibitory effects on the PDGFRβ.

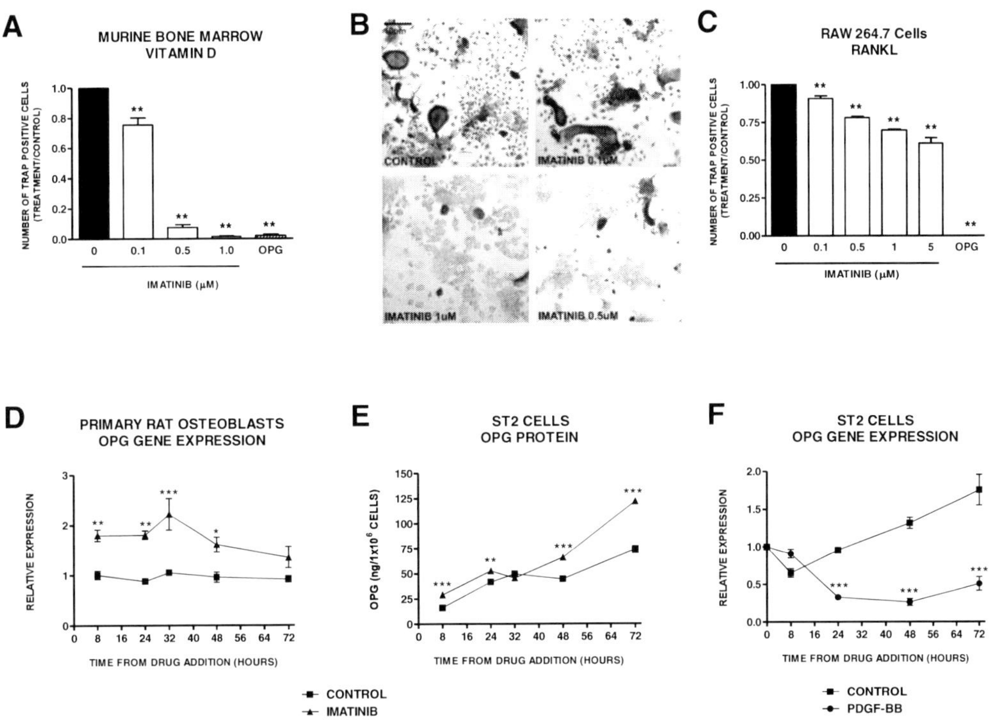

Figure 3. Effects of imatinib on osteoclastogenesis in A and B, murine bone marrow cultures treated with $1,25(OH)D_3$, and C, RAW-264.7 cells treated with RANKL 30ng/ml. D), Effect of imatinib on expression of OPG mRNA in primary rat osteoblasts. Gene expression is expressed relative to the 8 hour control value. E) Effect of imatinib on production of OPG protein by ST2 cells. F) Effect of PDGF-BB on expression of OPG mRNA. Gene expression is expressed relative to the 0 hour control value. Data are mean ± SEM. *, $p<0.05$ vs control; **, $p<0.01$ vs control; ***, $p<0.001$ vs control [72]. Reproduced with permission of American Society for Bone and Mineral Research.

As evidenced by its inhibitory effect in stromal-cell independent cultures [72], there may also be a direct effect of imatinib on osteoclastogenesis. The mechanism(s) by which imatinib directly inhibits osteoclastogenesis is uncertain. The proliferation and differentiation of osteoclast precursors (primary human monocyte/macrophage lineage cells) are inhibited by imatinib at doses of 0.3 to 3 μM [68]. PDGF-BB and PDGF-AA increases osteoclast number and function [51, 52, 88](O'Sullivan, manuscript in preparation), and therefore inhibition of the PDGFR(s) may underlie imatinib's direct effects on osteoclasts. However, these effects have been seen in stromal-cell dependent cultures (murine bone marrow or fetal rat calvaria), and PDGF-BB did not stimulate osteoclastogenesis in stromal cell-independent RANKL-treated RAW-264.7 cells. SCF has been shown to stimulate osteoclast formation and activity at high doses (1μg/ml) or in long term cultures [60, 61] but to have no effect at lower doses and shorter term cultures [72]. SCF mutant mice (*Sl/Sl^d*), lacking the membrane-bound form of SCF, have an increase in late stage osteoclast precursors [62]. In contrast, osteoclast development and function is normal in c-abl-null mice [47]. 1-3 μM imatinib significantly decreases RANK expression in CD14+ cells, and it was hypothesized that this effect is attributable to inhibition of c-fms, as RANK expression by osteoclasts is stimulated by M-CSF [105]. Imatinib has been shown to reduce M-CSF-induced inhibition of osteoclast apoptosis and M-CSF-induced bone resorption [83]. c-fms is inhibited by levels of imatinib (1.42μM) [70] that reduce osteoclastogenesis formation and activity in human CD14+ peripheral blood mononuclear cells [69]. Given the role of M-CSF in osteoclastogenesis [65, 106] it has been proposed that inhibition of c-fms mediates some of imatinib's direct effects on osteoclast formation and function [69, 107].

Taken as a whole, these data demonstrate that imatinib is a potent inhibitor of osteoclastogenesis and bone resorption, and promotes osteoclast apoptosis, *in vitro*. The mechanisms of these effects include an indirect effect through a reduction in stromal cell number, as well as through stromal cell production of regulatory cytokines, and a direct effect on osteoclast precursors and mature osteoclasts, as a result of inhibition of one or more of imatinib's target TKIs (Figure 4).

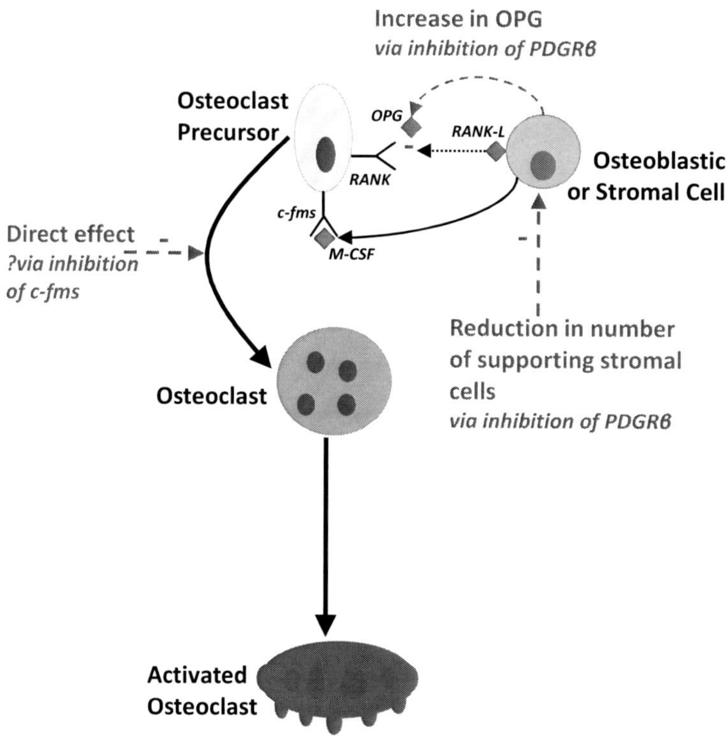

Figure 4. Effects and proposed mechanisms underlying effects of imatinib on osteoclastogenesis.

Animal Studies of Imatinib

Studies of imatinib's skeletal actions in humans have been either retrospective [79], cross-sectional [76, 79, 82], or uncontrolled [78, 81], and are potentially confounded by the effects of recovery from serious underlying illness. Studies in laboratory animals provide an opportunity to prospectively examine the skeletal actions of imatinib in a disease-free model. In a 5 week assessment of the skeletal effects of imatinib in healthy rats, there was a decrease in trabecular bone volume. This finding was accompanied by a reduction in serum osteocalcin, a marker of bone formation, and a reduction in osteoblast surface, as assessed by histomorphometry [75]. There was no evidence for an anti-resorptive action of imatinib, by either biochemical or histomorphometric assessment. In contrast, in collagen-induced arthritis (CIA) rats treated with imatinib mesylate for 4 weeks from the onset of arthritis, osteoclast formation was reduced [66]. In adult Balb/c mice treated with imatinib for 8 weeks there was a decrease in osteoclast activity but not osteoclast number [69]. Thus, there is evidence from animal studies for an inhibitory effect of imatinib on bone formation, osteoblast number and osteoclast number and function.

Effects of Imatinib in Adults

Several studies have evaluated the effects of imatinib on bone and calcium metabolism in humans. The most consistent effects of imatinib in these studies are the alterations in calcium and phosphate metabolism. Hypophosphatemia was noted in up to 50% of patients undergoing clinical trials with imatinib [15, 84]. In a cross-sectional analysis Berman et al found that 25 out of 49 patients being treated with imatinib for CML, GIST or sarcoma had hypophosphatemia [80]. All patients being treated with imatinib (with normal or low phosphate) had an increase in renal phosphate excretion, but those with hypophosphatemia also had lower serum calcium and high parathyroid hormone (PTH) levels. These results have been reiterated in other cross-sectional and retrospective studies [76, 77, 79, 82]. We have conducted the only prospective study of bone and calcium metabolism in patients receiving imatinib therapy. In this study of patients with CML, short term treatment with imatinib led to a mild secondary hyperparathyroidism [81] and extended follow-up demonstrates that this effect persists out to 48 months, but does not progress [78, 108] (Figure 4A-D) (Table 1). In a prospective study of patients receiving imatinib for GIST the majority of patients had phosphate levels below the normal range on at least one occasion during treatment, and most had lower mean plasma phosphate levels during treatment than at baseline [86]. In this and Berman's study, phosphate levels rose on stopping imatinib [80, 86]. In addition to the effects on calcium and phosphate metabolism, imatinib therapy is associated with altered bone remodelling. Thus, in prospectively collected data in patients with CML, initiation of imatinib led to an initial (<6mo) increase in markers of bone formation, without significant change in bone resorption [81]. With longer term treatment, markers of both bone formation and resorption fell, despite the persistence of mild secondary hyperparathyroidism, with changes persisting (but not worsening) to 4 years of treatment [78, 108] (Figure 4E and F) (Table 1). In cross-sectional studies, in which patients had been exposed to a variable duration of imatinib therapy for treatment of CML, GIST or sarcoma, levels of markers of bone turnover were generally low [76, 80, 82]. The initial increase in bone formation would be consistent with the finding that that imatinib promotes osteoblast differentiation *in vitro* [71-74, 79]. The fall in bone turnover during long-term therapy is consistent with imatinib's potent inhibition of osteoblast proliferation and osteoclastogenesis *in vitro* [66-69, 71-74, 79].

A proposed mechanism for the initial changes in calcium and phosphate metabolism is that the early increase in bone formation upon initiating imatinib may produce a net flux of calcium from extracellular fluid into bone, a fall in serum calcium, and a compensatory rise in the level of PTH, which acts to restore the serum calcium level. The development of secondary hyperparathyroidism promotes phosphaturia and a decline in the serum phosphate. However, in the longer term, there is sustained and coupled reduction in bone turnover, and the cause of the persistent secondary hyperparathyroidism in this light is unclear. In general, secondary hyperparathyroidism is not observed during long-term therapy with other drugs that reduce bone turnover [109]. It is possible that imatinib might directly affect renal tubular phosphate reabsorption, independent of changes in PTH. There has been one case report of partial Fanconi syndrome associated with imatinib therapy [110] and a report of massive aminoaciduria [111], but our prospective study did not find evidence of generalized proximal renal tubule dysfunction or changes in circulating levels of the phosphatonin FGF-23 [78, 112]. Jönsson et al proposed that hypomagnesemia might contribute to the mild hypocalcemia observed in imatinib-treated patients [82], but hypomagnesemia causes hypocalcemia by inhibiting PTH production, and levels of PTH are increased during imatinib. A possibility that has not yet been addressed is that imatinib decreases intestinal calcium absorption, thereby inducing secondary hyperparathyroidism.

In light of the effects on calcium and phosphate metabolism and bone turnover, there is theoretical potential for an effect on bone mass. In our prospective assessment of patients receiving imatinib for treatment of CML, bone mineral density (BMD) is stable or increased compared to baseline values at all sites (spine, proximal femur and total body) after 24 months and remained stable between 24 and 48 month (Figure 5A-C).

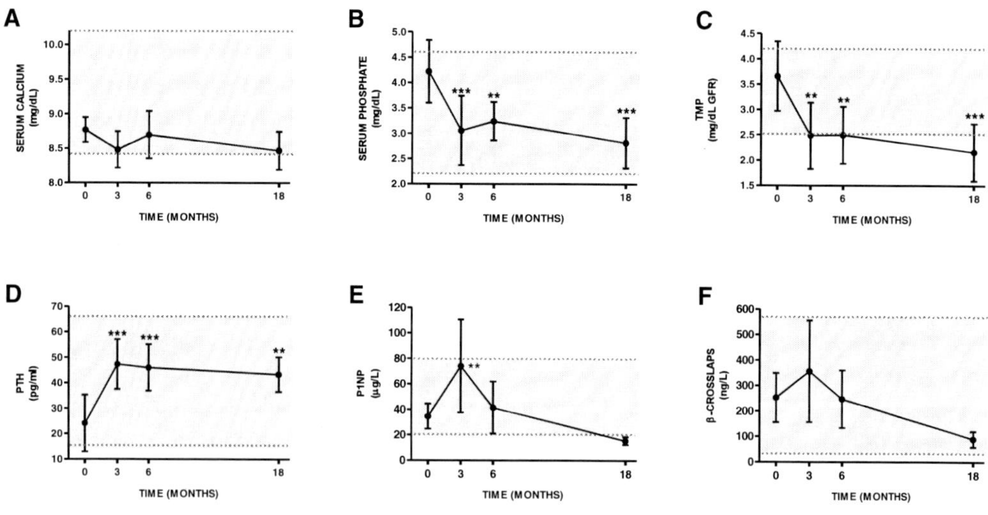

Figure 5. Biochemical measurements and levels of bone turnover in CML patients treated with imatinib. A, albumin-adjusted serum calcium; B, tubular maximum for phosphate reabsorption (TmP/GFR); C, serum phosphate; D, intact parathyroid hormone (PTH); E, serum procollagen type-I N-terminal propeptide (P1NP); F, serum β-C-terminal telopeptide of type I collagen (βCTX). Data are mean [95% CI]. **, p<0.01 vs baseline; ***, p<0.001 vs baseline. To convert to SI units: calcium, divide by 4; phosphate, divide by 3.1; TmP, divide by 3.1; PTH, divide by 9. The normal ranges are indicated by the shaded areas[78]. Copyright 2007, The Endocrine Society.

Table 1. Biochemical measurements and levels of bone turnover in CML patients treated with imatinib. TmP, tubular maximum for phosphate reabsorption ; PTH, intact parathyroid hormone; P1NP, serum procollagen type-I N-terminal propeptide; βCTX, serum β-C-terminal telopeptide of type I collagen. Data are mean [95% CI]. **, p<0.01 vs baseline; ***, p<0.001 vs baseline. To convert to SI units: calcium, divide by 4; phosphate, divide by 3.1; TmP, divide by 3.1; PTH, divide by 9. 18 month data are reproduced for illustrative purposes

	Change from Baseline	
	24 Months	**48 Months**
Serum Calcium (mg/dL)	8.5 (8.2, 8.7)	8.5 (8.3, 8.7)
Serum Phosphate (mg/dL)	2.8 (2.3, 3.3)***	3.2 (2.7, 3.6)***
TmP (mg/dL GFR)	1.8 (0.9, 2.5)***	2.2 (1.7, 2.7)***
PTH (pg/mL)	43.3 (37.0, 49.7)**	42.6 (32.6, 52.5)**
P1NP (μg/L)	15.6 (0, 30.9)*	21.4 (14.7, 28.1)
βCTX (ng/L)	93.0 (0, 194.5)	131.4 (93.9, 169)

These results are in keeping with cross-sectional studies showing well-preserved BMD or increased bone volume in patients treated with imatinib [76, 79, 82]. It is possible that direct effects of imatinib to initially increase bone formation and later decrease bone turnover contribute to the positive effects on BMD. However, other mechanisms, such as recovery from disease and the effects of increased body weight, which are known to be positive regulators of BMD [113], might also contribute. Significant increases have been observed in body weight and fat mass during imatinib therapy up to 24 months of treatment , with stability thereafter, well after the symptomatic improvement that occurs in response to initiation of imatinib therapy [78, 108] (Figure 5D-E) (Table 2).

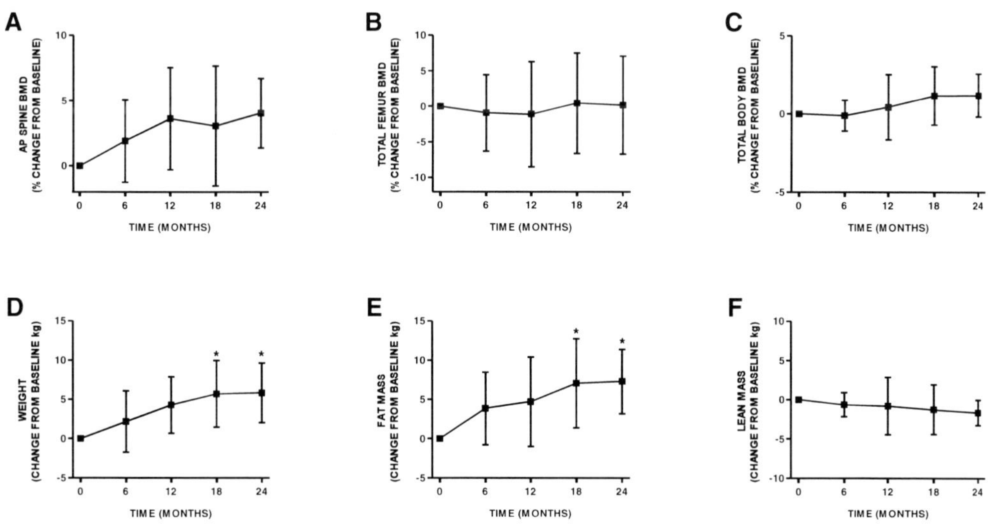

Figure 6. Bone density and body composition in CML patients treated with imatinib. A, Lumbar spine; B, Total femur; C, Total body; D, Weight; E, Fat mass; F, Lean mass. Data are mean [95% CI] percentage change from baseline (A-C) or mean [95% CI] change from baseline (D-F).*, p<0.05 vs baseline [78]. Copyright 2007, The Endocrine Society.

Table 2. Bone density and body composition in CML patients treated with imatinib.Data are mean [95% CI] percentage change from baseline for BMD or mean [95% CI] change in kg from baseline for weight, fat mass and lean mass.*p<0.05 vs baseline. 24 month data are reproduced for illustrative purposes.

	Change from Baseline	
	24 Months	**48 Months**
Lumbar Spine BMD	4.0 (1.4, 6.7)	3.1 (-0.2, 6.4)
Total Femur BMD	0.2 (-6.7, 7.1)	0.8 (-5, 6.5)
Total Body BMD	1.2 (-0.2, 2.6)	1.5 (-0.7, 3.6)
Weight	5.8 (2.0, 9.6)*	4.4 (1.0, 7.7)
Fat Mass	7.3 (3.2, 11.4)*	7.0 (4.3, 9.7)*
Lean Mass	-1.6 (-3.2, -0.1)	-3.4 (-6.0, -0.8)*

Effects of Imatinib in Children

In contrast to the neutral or positive effects of imatinib in adults there are case reports and retrospective case-series that report growth retardation in children receiving imatinib for treatment of CML [114-119]. Pre-pubertal children consistently demonstrated a reduction in height velocity (height standard deviation score (SDS) of between -0.5 and -1.5 SD) and this effect was apparent within months of starting imatinib. A recent review alluded to unpublished data from a prospective study of 22 children that showed similar effects within 12 months of treatment with imatinib [120]. Children who commenced imatinib pre-puberty regained (some) growth velocity upon entering puberty. In children who had entered puberty prior to starting imatinib there was, at most, only mild growth impairment [114-119]. Alterations in cartilage metabolism may explain this effect. *In vivo*, 9 month old rats treated with imatinib had a significant reduction in the width of the growth plate, and this was attributed to an inhibitory effect on chondrocyte proliferation and activity. It was proposed that this leads to reduced longitudinal bone growth and may underlie growth retardation in children treated with imatinib [121]. Alternatively, low levels of IGF1 have been observed in children [118, 122] and adults [123] treated with imatinib, and impaired growth has been attributed to acquired growth hormone (GH) deficiency.

A recent review alluded to unpublished data from a prospective study of 41 children treated with imatinib. In this study 25% developed hyperparathyroidism, levels of the bone resorption marker C-terminal cross-linking telopeptide of collagen type I (CTX) declined in 60% of the patients, while levels of osteocalcin were elevated at the beginning of treatment but declined to normal levels with continued treatment [120]. Similar changes in markers of bone turnover have been reported in cross-sectional analyses [114, 118]. There has not been any systematic evaluation of BMD, but there is a single case report of low BMD for chronological age in a 15 year old boy treated with imatinib for CML [114].

Although CML is uncommon in children, these emerging data suggest that imatinib therapy might have important effects on the growing skeleton. Careful clinical studies should be conducted in children and adolescents treated with imatinib.

Skeletal Effects of Related Tyrosine Kinase Inhibitors

In addition to imatinib, a number of related small molecule TKIs are emerging as effective treatments for CML. Nilotinib and dasatinib inhibit similar molecular targets to imatinib, although are more potent inhibitors of bcr-abl than imatinib, and dasatinib also targets c-src [25, 124-129]. Both agents are used to treat patients who are resistant or intolerant to treatment with imatinib [125, 130-136], but may assume an increased prominence in management of CML in the face of evidence they are superior to imatinib in achieving remission in patients with newly diagnosed CML [132, 137, 138]. Nilotinib is currently being investigated as a treatment for GIST [139-141] and dasatinib is undergoing preclinical trials for use in a number of malignant conditions [142]. Both agents have been reported to induce hypophosphatemia [132, 138, 143]. In a cross-sectional study, patients receiving nilotinib for treatment of CML because of imatinib-resistance or intolerance had a similar biochemical profile, with secondary hyperparathyroidism and reduced levels of bone turnover markers, to that observed in patients treated with imatinib [90]. BMD tended to be higher than normal in the nilotinib-treated group [90]. There are no similar studies in patients receiving dasatinib, however, in healthy mice or rats, treatment with dasatinib led to an increase in femora or tibia trabecular bone volume [144, 145] but not whole body BMD [145]. The increased BMD induced by dasatinib therapy has been variably attributed to an anti-resorptive effect [145] or an anabolic effect [144].

In a similar fashion to imatinib, nilotinib inhibits osteoclast formation and function, and promotes osteoclast apoptosis [90, 126]. Dasatinib has been shown to inhibit human, rat and murine osteoclast formation and activity *in vitro* and these effects have been attributed to inhibition of c-fms [145-147]. In osteoblasts, nilotinib inhibits osteoblast proliferation without affecting cell viability, mediated through inhibition of PDGFR signalling. In contrast to imatinib, nilotinib inhibits or has a neutral effect on osteoblast differentiation [90]. Dasatinib inhibits osteoblast proliferation [144, 145, 148-150]- an effect that has been attributed to inhibition of PDGFR [145] or of c-src [148]. While some authors report that dasatinib increases osteoblast differentiation [144, 148, 149, 151], others have found inhibition of osteoblast differentiation [150]. The putative target(s) for these actions include c-src, c-abl or PDGFR [148, 150, 151].

Bosutinib is a newer TKI, with activity restricted to c-src and c-abl, which has been shown to have activity in chronic phase chronic myeloid leukemia after imatinib and dasatinib and/or nilotinib therapy failure [152]. Treatment with bosutinib is associated with hypophosphatemia [152]. In one study bosutinib did not affect expression of genes associated with osteoblast differentiation in hBM-MSCs [151]. Sunitinib has activity against vascular endothelial growth factor receptors (VEGFR-1 and VEGFR-2), fetal liver tyrosine kinase receptor 3 (FLT3), c-kit, PDGFRα, and PDGFRβ in both biochemical and cellular assays [153-155], and has been approved for patients with advanced renal cell carcinoma (RCC) and GIST after disease progression or intolerance to imatinib mesylate therapy [156]. Treatment with sunitinib has been shown to lead to secondary hyperparathyroidism, although hypophosphatemia was much less common than was reported with imatinib and nilotinib [157]. These observations demonstrate that the effects observed on bone cells and bone and mineral metabolism are not unique to imatinib, and imply a role for one or more of the targets shared by imatinib and the second generation TKIs in mediating these effects.

Conclusion

Small molecule TKIs are emerging as powerful tools in the management of a variety of malignant and proliferative conditions. "Off target" effects have been observed with all these TKIs [15, 39-44, 129, 136, 158-161], including effects on bone and calcium metabolism [66-86, 108, 144-151]. Imatinib has potent effects on osteoblast and osteoclast formation and activity *in vitro* [66-69, 71-74, 79, 83] and this is consistent with its effects on bone turnover in patients with CML or GIST [76, 78, 80-82, 108]. In these patients, imatinib leads to secondary hyperparathyroidism and, in some cases, mild hypophosphatemia [76-82, 86, 108]. The similar effects on calcium and phosphate metabolism and PTH levels observed during treatment with related TKIs [90, 132, 138, 143, 152, 157] suggest that the mechanism relates to a common target kinase. The PDGFR is strongly implicated as a critical regulator of imatinib's *in vitro* effects [48, 72, 88, 89, 91, 92], although the effects on osteoclastogenesis may also be mediated via inhibition of c-fms, and one or both of these targets may play a role in mediating the clinical effects of imatinib on calcium and phosphate metabolism.

Despite the potential for deleterious effects on the skeleton, in adult humans imatinib has a positive effect on bone mass, and data are largely reassuring regarding the skeletal safety of short or long-term use of imatinib for treatment of CML or GIST [76, 78, 79, 81, 82, 108]. In children, there may be negative effects on growth [114-119, 162], and this possibility deserves additional research to understand its nature, magnitude and mechanism. Some authors recommend periodic monitoring of calcium and phosphate metabolism in patients receiving imatinib [82, 163]. The current data do not suggest a need to monitor BMD in these patients. Future studies aimed at elucidating the mechanisms of the cellular and clinical effects of imatinib and the related TKIs on bone and mineral metabolism will contribute to a greater understanding of the 'off-target' effects of these agents, and may provide an improved understanding of the mechanisms that regulate bone metabolism.

References

[1] Deininger M, Buchdunger E, Druker BJ. The development of imatinib as a therapeutic agent for chronic myeloid leukemia. *Blood.* 2005;105(7):2640-53.

[2] Druker BJ, Talpaz M, Resta DJ, Peng B, Buchdunger E, Ford JM, et al. Efficacy and safety of a specific inhibitor of the BCR-ABL tyrosine kinase in chronic myeloid leukemia. *N. Engl. J. Med.* 2001;344(14):1031-7.

[3] Druker BJ, Sawyers CL, Kantarjian H, Resta DJ, Reese SF, Ford JM, et al. Activity of a specific inhibitor of the BCR-ABL tyrosine kinase in the blast crisis of chronic myeloid leukemia and acute lymphoblastic leukemia with the Philadelphia chromosome. *N. Engl. J. Med.* 2001 Apr 5;344(14):1038-42.

[4] Kantarjian HM, Talpaz M, O'Brien S, Smith TL, Giles FJ, Faderl S, et al. Imatinib mesylate for Philadelphia chromosome-positive, chronic-phase myeloid leukemia after failure of interferon-alpha: follow-up results. *Clin. Cancer Res.* 2002;8(7):2177-87.

[5] Sawyers CL, Hochhaus A, Feldman E, Goldman JM, Miller CB, Ottmann OG, et al. Imatinib induces hematologic and cytogenetic responses in patients with chronic myelogenous leukemia in myeloid blast crisis: results of a phase II study. *Blood.* 2002 May 15;99(10):3530-9.

[6] Talpaz M, Silver RT, Druker BJ, Goldman JM, Gambacorti-Passerini C, Guilhot F, et al. Imatinib induces durable hematologic and cytogenetic responses in patients with accelerated phase chronic myeloid leukemia: results of a phase 2 study. *Blood.* 2002;99(6):1928-37.

[7] Baccarani M, Rosti G, de Vivo A, Bonifazi F, Russo D, Martinelli G, et al. A randomized study of interferon-alpha versus interferon-alpha and low-dose arabinosyl cytosine in chronic myeloid leukemia. *Blood.* 2002;99(5):1527-35.

[8] Guilhot F, Chastang C, Michallet M, Guerci A, Harousseau JL, Maloisel F, et al. Interferon alfa-2b combined with cytarabine versus interferon alone in chronic myelogenous leukemia. French Chronic Myeloid Leukemia Study Group. *N Engl. J. Med.* 1997;337(4):223-9.

[9] Hochhaus A, O'Brien SG, Guilhot F, Druker BJ, Branford S, Foroni L, et al. Six-year follow-up of patients receiving imatinib for the first-line treatment of chronic myeloid leukemia. *Leukemia.* 2009 Jun;23(6):1054-61.

[10] Shah NP, Nicoll JM, Nagar B, Gorre ME, Paquette RL, Kuriyan J, et al. Multiple BCR-ABL kinase domain mutations confer polyclonal resistance to the tyrosine kinase inhibitor imatinib (STI571) in chronic phase and blast crisis chronic myeloid leukemia. *Cancer Cell.* 2002;2(2):117-25.

[11] Gorre ME, Mohammed M, Ellwood K, Hsu N, Paquette R, Rao PN, et al. Clinical resistance to STI-571 cancer therapy caused by BCR-ABL gene mutation or amplification. *Science.* 2001;293(5531):876-80.

[12] Apperley JF. Part I: mechanisms of resistance to imatinib in chronic myeloid leukaemia. *Lancet Oncol.* 2007 Nov;8(11):1018-29.

[13] Marin D, Bazeos A, Mahon FX, Eliasson L, Milojkovic D, Bua M, et al. Adherence is the critical factor for achieving molecular responses in patients with chronic myeloid leukemia who achieve complete cytogenetic responses on imatinib. *J. Clin. Oncol.* 2010 May 10;28(14):2381-8.

[14] Noens L, van Lierde MA, De Bock R, Verhoef G, Zachee P, Berneman Z, et al. Prevalence, determinants, and outcomes of nonadherence to imatinib therapy in patients with chronic myeloid leukemia: the ADAGIO study. *Blood.* 2009 May 28;113(22):5401-11.

[15] O'Brien SG, Guilhot F, Larson RA, Gathmann I, Baccarani M, Cervantes F, et al. Imatinib compared with interferon and low-dose cytarabine for newly diagnosed chronic-phase chronic myeloid leukemia. *N. Engl. J. Med.* 2003;348(11):994-1004.

[16] Darkow T, Henk HJ, Thomas SK, Feng W, Baladi JF, Goldberg GA, et al. Treatment interruptions and non-adherence with imatinib and associated healthcare costs: a retrospective analysis among managed care patients with chronic myelogenous leukaemia. *Pharmacoeconomics.* 2007;25(6):481-96.

[17] Hughes TP, Kaeda J, Branford S, Rudzki Z, Hochhaus A, Hensley ML, et al. Frequency of major molecular responses to imatinib or interferon alfa plus cytarabine in newly diagnosed chronic myeloid leukemia. *N. Engl. J. Med.* 2003 Oct 9;349(15):1423-32.

[18] Mahon FX, Rea D, Guilhot J, Guilhot F, Huguet F, Nicolini F, et al. Discontinuation of imatinib in patients with chronic myeloid leukaemia who have maintained complete molecular remission for at least 2 years: the prospective, multicentre Stop Imatinib (STIM) trial. *Lancet Oncol.* 2010 Nov;11(11):1029-35.

[19] Buchdunger E, Cioffi CL, Law N, Stover D, Ohno-Jones S, Druker BJ, et al. Abl protein-tyrosine kinase inhibitor STI571 inhibits in vitro signal transduction mediated by c-kit and platelet-derived growth factor receptors. *J. Pharmacol Exp. Ther.* 2000;295(1):139-45.

[20] Buchdunger E, Zimmermann J, Mett H, Meyer T, Muller M, Druker BJ, et al. Inhibition of the Abl protein-tyrosine kinase in vitro and in vivo by a 2-phenylaminopyrimidine derivative. *Cancer Res.* 1996;56(1):100-4.

[21] Druker BJ, Tamura S, Buchdunger E, Ohno S, Segal GM, Fanning S, et al. Effects of a selective inhibitor of the Abl tyrosine kinase on the growth of Bcr-Abl positive cells. *Nat. Med.* 1996;2(5):561-6.

[22] Buchdunger E, Zimmermann J, Mett H, Meyer T, Muller M, Regenass U, et al. Selective inhibition of the platelet-derived growth factor signal transduction pathway by a protein-tyrosine kinase inhibitor of the 2-phenylaminopyrimidine class. *Proc. Natl. Acad. Sci. USA.* 1995;92(7):2558-62.

[23] Heinrich MC, Griffith DJ, Druker BJ, Wait CL, Ott KA, Zigler AJ. Inhibition of c-kit receptor tyrosine kinase activity by STI 571, a selective tyrosine kinase inhibitor. *Blood.* 2000;96(3):925-32.

[24] Dewar AL, Cambareri AC, Zannettino AC, Miller BL, Doherty KV, Hughes TP, et al. Macrophage colony-stimulating factor receptor c-fms is a novel target of imatinib. *Blood.* 2005;105(8):3127-32.

[25] Taylor JR, Brownlow N, Domin J, Dibb NJ. FMS receptor for M-CSF (CSF-1) is sensitive to the kinase inhibitor imatinib and mutation of Asp-802 to Val confers resistance. *Oncogene.* 2006;25(1):147-51.

[26] Verweij J, van Oosterom A, Blay JY, Judson I, Rodenhuis S, van der Graaf W, et al. Imatinib mesylate (STI-571 Glivec, Gleevec) is an active agent for gastrointestinal stromal tumours, but does not yield responses in other soft-tissue sarcomas that are unselected for a molecular target. Results from an EORTC Soft Tissue and Bone Sarcoma Group phase II study. *Eur. J. Cancer.* 2003;39(14):2006-11.

[27] Nilsson B, Sjolund K, Kindblom LG, Meis-Kindblom JM, Bumming P, Nilsson O, et al. Adjuvant imatinib treatment improves recurrence-free survival in patients with high-risk gastrointestinal stromal tumours (GIST). *Br. J. Cancer.* 2007 Jun 4;96(11):1656-8.

[28] Dematteo RP, Ballman KV, Antonescu CR, Maki RG, Pisters PW, Demetri GD, et al. Adjuvant imatinib mesylate after resection of localised, primary gastrointestinal stromal tumour: a randomised, double-blind, placebo-controlled trial. *Lancet.* 2009 Mar 28;373(9669):1097-104.

[29] Pisters PW, Colombo C. Adjuvant imatinib therapy for gastrointestinal stromal tumors. *J. Surg. Oncol.* 2011 Dec;104(8):896-900.

[30] Cools J, DeAngelo DJ, Gotlib J, Stover EH, Legare RD, Cortes J, et al. A tyrosine kinase created by fusion of the PDGFRA and FIP1L1 genes as a therapeutic target of

imatinib in idiopathic hypereosinophilic syndrome. *N. Engl. J. Med.* 2003;348(13):1201-14.

[31] Apperley JF, Gardembas M, Melo JV, Russell-Jones R, Bain BJ, Baxter EJ, et al. Response to imatinib mesylate in patients with chronic myeloproliferative diseases with rearrangements of the platelet-derived growth factor receptor beta. *N. Engl. J. Med.* 2002;347(7):481-7.

[32] David M, Cross NC, Burgstaller S, Chase A, Curtis C, Dang R, et al. Durable responses to imatinib in patients with PDGFRB fusion gene-positive and BCR-ABL-negative chronic myeloproliferative disorders. *Blood.* 2007 Jan 1;109(1):61-4.

[33] Boucher P, Gotthardt M, Li WP, Anderson RG, Herz J. LRP: role in vascular wall integrity and protection from atherosclerosis. *Science.* 2003;300(5617):329-32.

[34] Lassila M, Allen TJ, Cao Z, Thallas V, Jandeleit-Dahm KA, Candido R, et al. Imatinib attenuates diabetes-associated atherosclerosis. *Arterioscler Thromb. Vasc. Biol.* 2004;24(5):935-42.

[35] Gottardi M, Manzato E, Gherlinzoni F. Imatinib and hyperlipidemia. *N. Engl J. Med.* 2005;353(25):2722-3.

[36] Veneri D, Franchini M, Bonora E. Imatinib and regression of type 2 diabetes. *N Engl J Med.* 2005;352(10):1049-50.

[37] Paniagua RT, Sharpe O, Ho PP, Chan SM, Chang A, Higgins JP, et al. Selective tyrosine kinase inhibition by imatinib mesylate for the treatment of autoimmune arthritis. *J. Clin. Invest.* 2006;116(10):2633-42.

[38] Daniels CE, Wilkes MC, Edens M, Kottom TJ, Murphy SJ, Limper AH, et al. Imatinib mesylate inhibits the profibrogenic activity of TGF-beta and prevents bleomycin-mediated lung fibrosis. *J. Clin. Invest.* 2004;114(9):1308-16.

[39] Gambacorti-Passerini C, Tornaghi L, Cavagnini F, Rossi P, Pecori-Giraldi F, Mariani L, et al. Gynaecomastia in men with chronic myeloid leukaemia after imatinib. *Lancet.* 2003;361(9373):1954-6.

[40] Savage DG, Antman KH. Imatinib mesylate--a new oral targeted therapy. *N. Engl. J. Med.* 2002 Feb 28;346(9):683-93.

[41] Tsao AS, Kantarjian H, Cortes J, O'Brien S, Talpaz M. Imatinib mesylate causes hypopigmentation in the skin. *Cancer.* 2003;98(11):2483-7.

[42] Kerkela R, Grazette L, Yacobi R, Iliescu C, Patten R, Beahm C, et al. Cardiotoxicity of the cancer therapeutic agent imatinib mesylate. *Nat. Med.* 2006;12(8):908-16.

[43] Cross TJ, Bagot C, Portmann B, Wendon J, Gillett D. Imatinib mesylate as a cause of acute liver failure. *Am. J. Hematol.* 2006 Mar;81(3):189-92.

[44] Agostino NM, Chinchilli VM, Lynch CJ, Koszyk-Szewczyk A, Gingrich R, Sivik J, et al. Effect of the tyrosine kinase inhibitors (sunitinib, sorafenib, dasatinib, and imatinib) on blood glucose levels in diabetic and nondiabetic patients in general clinical practice. *J. Oncol Pharm Pract.* 2011 Sep;17(3):197-202.

[45] Muller R, Slamon DJ, Tremblay JM, Cline MJ, Verma IM. Differential expression of cellular oncogenes during pre- and postnatal development of the mouse. *Nature.* 1982 Oct 14;299(5884):640-4.

[46] O'Neill AJ, Cotter TG, Russell JM, Gaffney EF. Abl expression in human fetal and adult tissues, tumours, and tumour microvessels. *J. Pathol.* 1997 Nov;183(3):325-9.

[47] Li B, Boast S, de los Santos K, Schieren I, Quiroz M, Teitelbaum SL, et al. Mice deficient in Abl are osteoporotic and have defects in osteoblast maturation. *Nat. Genet.* 2000;24(3):304-8.
[48] Chaudhary LR, Hofmeister AM, Hruska KA. Differential growth factor control of bone formation through osteoprogenitor differentiation. *Bone.* 2004;34(3):402-11.
[49] Kim HD, Valentini RF. Human osteoblast response in vitro to platelet-derived growth factor and transforming growth factor-beta delivered from controlled-release polymer rods. *Biomaterials.* 1997;18(17):1175-84.
[50] Okazaki R, Ikeda K, Sakamoto A, Nakano T, Morimoto K, Kikuchi T, et al. Transcriptional activation of c-fos and c-jun protooncogenes by serum growth factors in osteoblast-like MC3T3-E1 cells. *J. Bone Miner Res.* 1992;7(10):1149-55.
[51] Cochran DL, Rouse CA, Lynch SE, Graves DT. Effects of platelet-derived growth factor isoforms on calcium release from neonatal mouse calvariae. *Bone.* 1993;14(1):53-8.
[52] Zhang Z, Chen J, Jin D. Platelet-derived growth factor (PDGF)-BB stimulates osteoclastic bone resorption directly: the role of receptor beta. *Biochem. Biophys. Res. Commun.* 1998;251(1):190-4.
[53] Soriano P. The PDGF alpha receptor is required for neural crest cell development and for normal patterning of the somites. *Development.* 1997;124(14):2691-700.
[54] Bostrom H, Willetts K, Pekny M, Leveen P, Lindahl P, Hedstrand H, et al. PDGF-A signaling is a critical event in lung alveolar myofibroblast development and alveogenesis. *Cell.* 1996;85(6):863-73.
[55] Soriano P. Abnormal kidney development and hematological disorders in PDGF beta-receptor mutant mice. *Genes Dev.* 1994;8(16):1888-96.
[56] Leveen P, Pekny M, Gebre-Medhin S, Swolin B, Larsson E, Betsholtz C. Mice deficient for PDGF B show renal, cardiovascular, and hematological abnormalities. *Genes Dev.* 1994;8(16):1875-87.
[57] Mitlak BH, Finkelman RD, Hill EL, Li J, Martin B, Smith T, et al. The effect of systemically administered PDGF-BB on the rodent skeleton. *J. Bone Miner Res.* 1996;11(2):238-47.
[58] Nash TJ, Howlett CR, Martin C, Steele J, Johnson KA, Hicklin DJ. Effect of platelet-derived growth factor on tibial osteotomies in rabbits. *Bone.* 1994;15(2):203-8.
[59] Gattei V, Aldinucci D, Quinn JM, Degan M, Cozzi M, Perin V, et al. Human osteoclasts and preosteoclast cells (FLG 29.1) express functional c-kit receptors and interact with osteoblast and stromal cells via membrane-bound stem cell factor. *Cell Growth Differ.* 1996;7(6):753-63.
[60] van't Hof RJ, von Lindern M, Nijweide PJ, Beug H. Stem cell factor stimulates chicken osteoclast activity in vitro. *FASEB J.* 1997;11(4):287-93.
[61] Demulder A, Suggs SV, Zsebo KM, Scarcez T, Roodman GD. Effects of stem cell factor on osteoclast-like cell formation in long-term human marrow cultures. *J. Bone Miner Res.* 1992;7(11):1337-44.
[62] Lotinun S, Evans GL, Turner RT, Oursler MJ. Deletion of membrane-bound steel factor results in osteopenia in mice. *J. Bone Miner Res.* 2005;20(4):644-52.
[63] Ross FP. M-CSF, c-Fms, and signaling in osteoclasts and their precursors. *Ann. NY Acad. Sci.* 2006;1068:110-6.

[64] Fixe P, Praloran V. M-CSF: haematopoietic growth factor or inflammatory cytokine? *Cytokine.* 1998;10(1):32-7.

[65] Yoshida H, Hayashi S, Kunisada T, Ogawa M, Nishikawa S, Okamura H, et al. The murine mutation osteopetrosis is in the coding region of the macrophage colony stimulating factor gene. *Nature.* 1990;345(6274):442-4.

[66] Ando W, Hashimoto J, Nampei A, Tsuboi H, Tateishi K, Ono T, et al. Imatinib mesylate inhibits osteoclastogenesis and joint destruction in rats with collagen-induced arthritis (CIA). *J. Bone Miner Metab.* 2006;24(4):274-82.

[67] Dewar AL, Doherty KV, Hughes TP, Lyons AB. Imatinib inhibits the functional capacity of cultured human monocytes. *Immunol. Cell Biol.* 2005;83(1):48-56.

[68] Dewar AL, Domaschenz RM, Doherty KV, Hughes TP, Lyons AB. Imatinib inhibits the in vitro development of the monocyte/macrophage lineage from normal human bone marrow progenitors. *Leukemia.* 2003;17(9):1713-21.

[69] Dewar AL, Farrugia AN, Condina MR, Bik To L, Hughes TP, Vernon-Roberts B, et al. Imatinib as a potential antiresorptive therapy for bone disease. *Blood.* 2006;107(11):4334-7.

[70] Dewar AL, Zannettino AC, Hughes TP, Lyons AB. Inhibition of c-fms by imatinib: expanding the spectrum of treatment. *Cell Cycle.* 2005;4(7):851-3.

[71] Fierro F, Illmer T, Jing D, Schleyer E, Ehninger G, Boxberger S, et al. Inhibition of platelet-derived growth factor receptorb by imatinib mesylate suppresses proliferation and alters differentiation of human mesencymal stem cells *in vitro. Cell Prolif.* 2007;40:355-66.

[72] O'Sullivan S, Naot D, Callon K, Porteous F, Horne A, Wattie D, et al. Imatinib promotes osteoblast differentiation by inhibiting PDGFR signaling and inhibits osteoclastogenesis by both direct and stromal cell-dependent mechanisms. *J. Bone Miner Res.* 2007 Nov;22(11):1679-89.

[73] Tibullo D, Giallongo C, La Cava P, Berretta S, Stagno F, Chiarenza A, et al. Effects of imatinib mesylate in osteoblastogenesis. *Exp. Hematol.* 2009 Apr;37(4):461-8.

[74] Jonsson S, Hjorth-Hansen H, Olsson B, Wadenvik H, Sundan A, Standal T. Imatinib inhibits proliferation of human mesenchymal stem cells and promotes early but not late osteoblast differentiation in vitro. *J. Bone Miner Metab.* 2012;30(1):119-23.

[75] O'Sullivan S, Naot D, Callon K, Watson M, Gamble G, Ladefoged M, et al. Imatinib mesylate does not increase bone volume in vivo. *Calcif Tissue Int.* 2011;88(1):16-22.

[76] Jonsson S, Olsson B, Ohlsson C, Lorentzon M, Mellstrom D, Wadenvik H. Increased cortical bone mineralization in imatinib treated patients with chronic myelogenous leukemia. *Haematologica.* 2008;93(7):1101-3.

[77] Osorio S, Garcia Noblejas A, Duran A, Steegmann J. Imatinib Mesylate Induces Hypophosphatemia in Patients With Chronic Myeloid Leukemia in Late Chronic Phase, and This Effect is Associated With Response. *Am. J. Hematol.* 2007;82.

[78] O'Sullivan S, Horne A, Wattie D, Porteous F, Callon K, Gamble G, et al. Decreased bone turnover despite persistent secondary hyperparathyroidism during prolonged treatment with imatinib. *J. Clin. Endocrinol. Metab.* 2009;94(4):1131-6.

[79] Fitter S, Dewar AL, Kostakis P, To LB, Hughes TP, Roberts MM, et al. Long-term imatinib therapy promotes bone formation in CML patients. *Blood.* 2008 Mar 1;111(5):2538-47.

[80] Berman E, Nicolaides M, Maki RG, Fleisher M, Chanel S, Scheu K, et al. Altered bone and mineral metabolism in patients receiving imatinib mesylate. *N. Engl. J. Med.* 2006;354(19):2006-13.

[81] Grey A, O'Sullivan S, Reid IR, Browett P. Imatinib mesylate, increased bone formation, and secondary hyperparathyroidism. *N. Engl. J. Med.* 2006;355(23):2494-5.

[82] Jonsson S, Standal T, Olsson B, Mellstrom D, Wadenvik H. Secondary hyperparathyroidism but stable bone-mineral density in patients with chronic myeloid leukemia treated with imatinib. *Am. J. Hematol.* 2012;87(5):550-2.

[83] El Hajj Dib I, Gallet M, Mentaverri R, Sevenet N, Brazier M, Kamel S. Imatinib mesylate (Gleevec) enhances mature osteoclast apoptosis and suppresses osteoclast bone resorbing activity. *Eur. J. Pharmacol.* 2006;551(1-3):27-33.

[84] Owen S, Hatfield A, Letvak L. Imatinib and altered bone and mineral metabolism. *N Engl. J. Med.* 2006;355(6):627.

[85] Gallet M, Mentaverri R, Sevenet N, Brazier M, Kamel S. Ability of breast cancer cell lines to stimulate bone resorbing activity of mature osteoclasts correlates with an anti-apoptotic effect mediated by macrophage colony stimulating factor. *Apoptosis.* 2006 Nov;11(11):1909-21.

[86] Joensuu H, Reichardt P. Imatinib and altered bone and mineral metabolism. *N. Engl. J. Med.* 2006;355(6):628.

[87] Aubin JE, Lian JB, Stein GS. Bone formation: maturation and functional activities of osteoblast lineage cells. In: Favus MJ, editor. Primer on the Metabolic Bone Diseases and Disorders of Mineral Metabolism. Washington, D.C.: *American Society for Bone and Mineral Research*; 2006. p. 20-9.

[88] Hock JM, Canalis E. Platelet-derived growth factor enhances bone cell replication, but not differentiated function of osteoblasts. *Endocrinology.* 1994;134(3):1423-8.

[89] Canalis E, McCarthy TL, Centrella M. Effects of platelet-derived growth factor on bone formation in vitro. *J. Cell Physiol.* 1989;140(3):530-7.

[90] O'Sullivan S, Lin J-M, Watson M, Callon K, Tong PC, Naot D, et al. The skeletal effects of the tyrosine kinase inhibitor nilotinib. *Bone.* 2011;49(2):281-9.

[91] Tokunaga A, Oya T, Ishii Y, Motomura H, Nakamura C, Ishizawa S, et al. PDGF receptor beta is a potent regulator of mesenchymal stromal cell function. *J. Bone Miner Res.* 2008 Sep;23(9):1519-28.

[92] Yu X, Hsieh SC, Bao W, Graves DT. Temporal expression of PDGF receptors and PDGF regulatory effects on osteoblastic cells in mineralizing cultures. *Am. J. Physiol.* 1997;272(5 Pt 1):C1709-16.

[93] Ross FP. Osteoclast biology and bone resorption. In: Favus MJ, editor. Primer on the Metabolic Bone Diseases and Disorders of Mineral Metabolism. Washington, D.C.: *American Society for Bone and Mineral Research*; 2006. p. 30-5.

[94] Teitelbaum SL, Abu-Amer Y, Ross FP. Molecular mechanisms of bone resorption. *J. Cell Biochem.* 1995;59(1):1-10.

[95] Boyle WJ, Simonet WS, Lacey DL. Osteoclast differentiation and activation. *Nature.* 2003;423(6937):337-42.

[96] Suda T, Takahashi N, Udagawa N, Jimi E, Gillespie MT, Martin TJ. Modulation of osteoclast differentiation and function by the new members of the tumor necrosis factor receptor and ligand families. *Endocr. Rev.* 1999;20(3):345-57.

[97] Pixley FJ, Stanley ER. CSF-1 regulation of the wandering macrophage: complexity in action. *Trends Cell Biol.* 2004;14(11):628-38.

[98] Hofbauer LC, Heufelder AE. Role of receptor activator of nuclear factor-kappaB ligand and osteoprotegerin in bone cell biology. *J. Mol. Med.* 2001;79(5-6):243-53.

[99] Theill LE, Boyle WJ, Penninger JM. RANK-L and RANK: T cells, bone loss, and mammalian evolution. *Annu. Rev. Immunol.* 2002;20:795-823.

[100] Walsh MC, Choi Y. Biology of the TRANCE axis. *Cytokine Growth Factor Rev.* 2003;14(3-4):251-63.

[101] Simonet WS, Lacey DL, Dunstan CR, Kelley M, Chang MS, Luthy R, et al. Osteoprotegerin: a novel secreted protein involved in the regulation of bone density. *Cell.* 1997;89(2):309-19.

[102] Cohen MM, Jr. The new bone biology: pathologic, molecular, and clinical correlates. *American Journal of Medical Genetics Part A.* 2006;140(23):2646-706.

[103] Baron R. General principles of bone biology. In: Favus MJ, editor. Primer on the Metabolic Bone Diseases and Disorders of Mineral Metabolism. Washington, D.C.: *American Society for Bone and Mineral Research*; 2003. p. 1-8.

[104] Hofbauer LC, Khosla S, Dunstan CR, Lacey DL, Boyle WJ, Riggs BL. The roles of osteoprotegerin and osteoprotegerin ligand in the paracrine regulation of bone resorption. *J. Bone Miner Res.* 2000;15(1):2-12.

[105] Arai F, Miyamoto T, Ohneda O, Inada T, Sudo T, Brasel K, et al. Commitment and differentiation of osteoclast precursor cells by the sequential expression of c-Fms and receptor activator of nuclear factor kappaB (RANK) receptors. *J. Exp. Med.* 1999;190(12):1741-54.

[106] Hodge JM, Kirkland MA, Nicholson GC. Multiple roles of M-CSF in human osteoclastogenesis. *J Cell Biochem.* 2007;102(3):759-68.

[107] Vandyke K, Fitter S, Dewar AL, Hughes TP, Zannettino ACW. Dysregulation of bone remodeling by imatinib mesylate. *Blood.* 2010;115(4):766-74.

[108] O'Sullivan S, Horne A, Wattie D, Porteous F, Gamble G, Browett P, Grey A. Bone Metabolism During Long-term Treatment with Imatinib.*Leuk Lymphoma.* 2013 Jan 24 .

[109] McClung MR, Lewiecki EM, Cohen SB, Bolognese MA, Woodson GC, Moffett AH, et al. Denosumab in postmenopausal women with low bone mineral density. *N. Engl. J. Med.* 2006;354(8):821-31.

[110] Francois H, Coppo P, Hayman JP, Fouqueray B, Mougenot B, Ronco P. Partial fanconi syndrome induced by imatinib therapy: a novel cause of urinary phosphate loss. *Am. J. Kidney Dis.* 2008 Feb;51(2):298-301.

[111] Ianotto J-C, Tempescul A, Amet Y, Grall P, Dalbies F, Eveillard J-R, et al. Imatinib mesylate induces massive and nonspecific aminoaciduria in CML patients. *Am. J. Hematol.* 2012;87(4):437-9.

[112] Fukumoto S, Yamashita T. FGF23 is a hormone-regulating phosphate metabolism--unique biological characteristics of FGF23. *Bone.* 2007 May;40(5):1190-5.

[113] Reid IR. Relationships between fat and bone. *Osteoporos Int.* 2008;19(5):595-606.

[114] Mariani S, Giona F, Basciani S, Brama M, Gnessi L. Low bone density and decreased inhibin-B/FSH ratio in a boy treated with imatinib during puberty. *Lancet.* 2008;372(9633):111-2.

[115] Kimoto T, Inoue M, Kawa K. Growth deceleration in a girl treated with imatinib. *Int. J. Hematol.* 2009;89(2):251-2.

[116] Shima H, Tokuyama M, Tanizawa A, Tono C, Hamamoto K, Muramatsu H, et al. Distinct impact of imatinib on growth at prepubertal and pubertal ages of children with chronic myeloid leukemia. *J. Pediatr*. 2011;159(4):676-81.

[117] Bansal D, Shava U, Varma N, Trehan A, Marwaha RK. Imatinib has adverse effect on growth in children with chronic myeloid leukemia. *Pediatr Blood Cancer*. 2011 Nov 2.

[118] Schmid H, Jaeger BAS, Lohse J, Suttorp M. Longitudinal growth retardation in a prepuberal girl with chronic myeloid leukemia on long-term treatment with imatinib. *Haematologica*. 2009;94(8):1177-9.

[119] Rastogi MV, Stork L, Druker B, Blasdel C, Nguyen T, Boston BA. Imatinib mesylate causes growth deceleration in pediatric patients with chronic myelogenous leukemia. *Pediatr Blood Cancer*. 2012 Feb 29.

[120] Suttorp M, Yaniv I, Schultz KR. Controversies in the treatment of CML in children and adolescents: TKIs versus BMT? *Biol Blood Marrow Transplant*. 2011 Jan;17(1 Suppl):S115-22.

[121] Vandyke K, Dewar AL, Fitter S, Menicanin D, To LB, Hughes TP, et al. Imatinib mesylate causes growth plate closure in vivo. *Leukemia*. 2009 Nov;23(11):2155-9.

[122] Hobernicht SL, Schweiger B, Zeitler P, Wang M, Hunger SP. Acquired Growth Hormone Deficiency in a Girl With Chronic Myelogenous Leukemia Treated With Tyrosine Kinase Inhibitor Therapy. *Pediatr Blood Cancer*. 2011 Apr;56(4):671-3.

[123] Kebapcilar L, Bilgir O, Alacacioglu I, Payzin B, Bilgir F, Oner P, et al. Does imatinib mesylate therapy cause growth hormone deficiency? *Med. Princ Pract*. 2009;18(5):360-3.

[124] Weisberg E, Wright RD, Jiang J, Ray A, Moreno D, Manley PW, et al. Effects of PKC412, nilotinib, and imatinib against GIST-associated PDGFRA mutants with differential imatinib sensitivity. *Gastroenterology*. 2006;131(6):1734-42.

[125] Weisberg E, Manley PW, Breitenstein W, Bruggen J, Cowan-Jacob SW, Ray A, et al. Characterization of AMN107, a selective inhibitor of native and mutant Bcr-Abl. *Cancer Cell*. 2005 Feb;7(2):129-41.

[126] Brownlow N, Russell AE, Saravanapavan H, Wiesmann M, Murray JM, Manley PW, et al. Comparison of nilotinib and imatinib inhibition of FMS receptor signaling, macrophage production and osteoclastogenesis. *Leukemia*. 2008;22(3):649-52.

[127] Karaman MW, Herrgard S, Treiber DK, Gallant P, Atteridge CE, Campbell BT, et al. A quantitative analysis of kinase inhibitor selectivity. *Nat. Biotechnol*. 2008 Jan;26(1):127-32.

[128] Lombardo LJ, Lee FY, Chen P, Norris D, Barrish JC, Behnia K, et al. Discovery of N-(2-chloro-6-methyl-phenyl)-2-(6-(4-(2-hydroxyethyl)-piperazin-1-yl)-2-methylpyrimidin-4- ylamino)thiazole-5-carboxamide (BMS-354825), a dual Src/Abl kinase inhibitor with potent antitumor activity in preclinical assays. *J. Med. Chem*. 2004 Dec 30;47(27):6658-61.

[129] Kantarjian H, Jabbour E, Grimley J, Kirkpatrick P. Dasatinib. *Nat. Rev. Drug Discov*. 2006;5(9):717-8.

[130] Shah NP, Tran C, Lee FY, Chen P, Norris D, Sawyers CL. Overriding imatinib resistance with a novel ABL kinase inhibitor. *Science*. 2004;305(5682):399-401.

[131] Ray A, Cowan-Jacob SW, Manley PW, Mestan J, Griffin JD. Identification of BCR-ABL point mutations conferring resistance to the Abl kinase inhibitor AMN107 (nilotinib) by a random mutagenesis study. *Blood*. 2007;109(11):5011-5.

[132] Saglio G, Kim D-W, Issaragrisil S, le Coutre P, Etienne G, Lobo C, et al. Nilotinib versus imatinib for newly diagnosed chronic myeloid leukemia. *N. Engl. J. Med.* 2010;362(24):2251-9.
[133] O'Hare T, Walters DK, Stoffregen EP, Jia T, Manley PW, Mestan J, et al. In vitro activity of Bcr-Abl inhibitors AMN107 and BMS-354825 against clinically relevant imatinib-resistant Abl kinase domain mutants. *Cancer Res.* 2005;65(11):4500-5.
[134] Hochhaus A, Kantarjian HM, Baccarani M, Lipton JH, Apperley JF, Druker BJ, et al. Dasatinib induces notable hematologic and cytogenetic responses in chronic-phase chronic myeloid leukemia after failure of imatinib therapy. *Blood.* 2007;109(6):2303-9.
[135] Talpaz M, Shah NP, Kantarjian H, Donato N, Nicoll J, Paquette R, et al. Dasatinib in imatinib-resistant Philadelphia chromosome-positive leukemias. *N. Engl. J. Med.* 2006;354(24):2531-41.
[136] Kantarjian H, Giles F, Wunderle L, Bhalla K, O'Brien S, Wassmann B, et al. Nilotinib in imatinib-resistant CML and Philadelphia chromosome-positive ALL. *N. Engl. J. Med.* 2006;354(24):2542-51.
[137] Kantarjian H, Shah NP, Hochhaus A, Cortes J, Shah S, Ayala M, et al. Dasatinib versus imatinib in newly diagnosed chronic-phase chronic myeloid leukemia. *N. Engl. J. Med.* 2010;362(24):2260-70.
[138] Kantarjian HM, Shah NP, Cortes JE, Baccarani M, Agarwal MB, Undurraga MS, et al. Dasatinib or imatinib in newly diagnosed chronic-phase chronic myeloid leukemia: 2-year follow-up from a randomized phase 3 trial (DASISION). *Blood.* 2012;119 (5):1123-9.
[139] Montemurro M, Schoffski P, Reichardt P, Gelderblom H, Schutte J, Hartmann JT, et al. Nilotinib in the treatment of advanced gastrointestinal stromal tumours resistant to both imatinib and sunitinib. *Eur. J. Cancer.* 2009;45(13):2293-7.
[140] Cauchi C, Somaiah N, Engstrom PF, Litwin S, Lopez M, Lee J, et al. Evaluation of nilotinib in advanced GIST previously treated with imatinib and sunitinib. *Cancer Chemother Pharmacol.* 2012;69(4):977-82.
[141] Reichardt P, Montemurro M. Clinical experience to date with nilotinib in gastrointestinal stromal tumors. *Semin. Oncol.* 2011;38 Suppl 1:S20-7.
[142] Gnoni A, Marech I, Silvestris N, Vacca A, Lorusso V. Dasatinib: an anti-tumour agent via Src inhibition. *Curr. Drug Targets.* 2011;12(4):563-78.
[143] Kantarjian HM, Giles FJ, Bhalla KN, Pinilla-Ibarz J, Larson RA, Gattermann N, et al. Nilotinib is effective in patients with chronic myeloid leukemia in chronic phase after imatinib resistance or intolerance: 24-month follow-up results. *Blood.* 2011;117(4):1141-5.
[144] Garcia-Gomez A, Ocio EM, Crusoe E, Santamaria C, Hernandez-Campo P, Blanco JF, et al. Dasatinib as a bone-modifying agent: anabolic and anti-resorptive effects. *PLoS One.* 2012;7(4):e34914.
[145] Vandyke K, Dewar AL, Diamond P, Fitter S, Schultz CG, Sims NA, et al. The tyrosine kinase inhibitor dasatinib dysregulates bone remodeling through inhibition of osteoclasts in vivo. *J. Bone Miner Res.* 2010 Aug;25(8):1759-70.
[146] Vandyke K, Dewar AL, Farrugia AN, Fitter S, Bik To L, Hughes TP, et al. Therapeutic concentrations of dasatinib inhibit in vitro osteoclastogenesis. *Leukemia.* 2009;23(5):994-7.

[147] Brownlow N, Mol C, Hayford C, Ghaem-Maghami S, Dibb NJ. Dasatinib is a potent inhibitor of tumour-associated macrophages, osteoclasts and the FMS receptor. *Leukemia.* 2009 Mar;23(3):590-4.
[148] Lee YC, Huang CF, Murshed M, Chu K, Araujo JC, Ye X, et al. Src family kinase/abl inhibitor dasatinib suppresses proliferation and enhances differentiation of osteoblasts. *Oncogene.* 2010 Jun 3;29(22):3196-207.
[149] Id Boufker H, Lagneaux L, Najar M, Piccart M, Ghanem G, Body JJ, et al. The Src inhibitor dasatinib accelerates the differentiation of human bone marrow-derived mesenchymal stromal cells into osteoblasts. *BMC Cancer.* 2010;10:298.
[150] Jonsson S, Hjorth-Hansen H, Olsson B, Wadenvik H, Sundan A, Standal T. Second-generation TKI dasatinib inhibits proliferation of mesenchymal stem cells and osteoblast differentiation in vitro. *Leukemia.* 2010 Jul;24(7):1357-9.
[151] Tibullo D, Barbagallo I, Giallongo C, La Cava P, Branca A, Conticello C, et al. Effects of second-generation tyrosine kinase inhibitors towards osteogenic differentiation of human mesenchymal cells of healthy donors. *Hematol. Oncol.* 2012 Mar;30(1):27-33.
[152] Khoury HJ, Cortes JE, Kantarjian HM, Gambacorti-Passerini C, Baccarani M, Kim D-W, et al. Bosutinib is active in chronic phase chronic myeloid leukemia after imatinib and dasatinib and/or nilotinib therapy failure. *Blood.* 2012;119(15):3403-12.
[153] Abrams TJ, Lee LB, Murray LJ, Pryer NK, Cherrington JM. SU11248 inhibits KIT and platelet-derived growth factor receptor beta in preclinical models of human small cell lung cancer. *Mol. Cancer Ther.* 2003;2(5):471-8.
[154] O'Farrell A-M, Abrams TJ, Yuen HA, Ngai TJ, Louie SG, Yee KWH, et al. SU11248 is a novel FLT3 tyrosine kinase inhibitor with potent activity in vitro and in vivo. *Blood.* 2003;101(9):3597-605.
[155] Mendel DB, Laird AD, Xin X, Louie SG, Christensen JG, Li G, et al. In vivo antitumor activity of SU11248, a novel tyrosine kinase inhibitor targeting vascular endothelial growth factor and platelet-derived growth factor receptors: determination of a pharmacokinetic/pharmacodynamic relationship. *Clin. Cancer Res.* 2003;9(1):327-37.
[156] Le Tourneau C, Raymond E, Faivre S. Sunitinib: a novel tyrosine kinase inhibitor. A brief review of its therapeutic potential in the treatment of renal carcinoma and gastrointestinal stromal tumors (GIST). *Ther Clin Risk Manag.* 2007;3(2):341-8.
[157] Baldazzi V, Tassi R, Lapini A, Lunghi A, Garofoli E, Caruso S, et al. Sunitinib-induced hyperparathyroidism: A possible mechanism to altered bone homeostasis. *Cancer.* 2012;118(12):3165-72.
[158] Zipfel PA, Zhang W, Quiroz M, Pendergast AM. Requirement for Abl kinases in T cell receptor signaling. *Curr. Biol.* 2004 Jul 27;14(14):1222-31.
[159] Steegman JL, Cervantes F, Le Coutre P, Porkka K, Saglio G. Off-target effects of BCR–ABL1 inhibitors and their potential long-term implications in patients with chronic myeloid leukemia. *Leuk Lymphoma.* 2012.
[160] Cortes JE, Kantarjian HM, Brummendorf TH, Kim DW, Turkina AG, Shen ZX, et al. Safety and efficacy of bosutinib (SKI-606) in chronic phase Philadelphia chromosome-positive chronic myeloid leukemia patients with resistance or intolerance to imatinib. *Blood.* 2011 Oct 27;118(17):4567-76.
[161] Morabito A, De Maio E, Di Maio M, Normanno N, Perrone F. Tyrosine kinase inhibitors of vascular endothelial growth factor receptors in clinical trials: current status and future directions. *Oncologist.* 2006 Jul-Aug;11(7):753-64.

[162] Millot F, Baruchel A, Guilhot J, Petit A, Leblanc T, Bertrand Y, et al. Imatinib is effective in children with previously untreated chronic myelogenous leukemia in early chronic phase: results of the French national phase IV trial. *J. Clin. Oncol.* 2011 Jul 10;29(20):2827-32.
[163] Atallah E, Kantarjian H, Cortes J. Emerging safety issues with imatinib and other Abl tyrosine kinase inhibitors. *Clin. Lymphoma Myeloma*. 2007;7 Suppl 3:S105-12.

In: Imatinib
Editors: Mojtaba Akhtari and Ihab Elhemaidi

ISBN: 978-1-62808-297-5

Chapter 7

Effects of Tyrosine Kinase Inhibitors on Growth in Pediatric Patients

Kate Vandyke and Andrew C.W. Zannettino
Myeloma Research Laboratory, Division of Haematology, Centre for Cancer Biology, SA Pathology and School of Medical Sciences, University of Adelaide, Adelaide, Australia

Abstract

Chronic myeloid leukemia (CML) is rarely seen in children, accounting for less than 3% of all childhood leukemias. Imatinib is currently recommended as a front-line therapy for chronic phase Ph+ CML in children and, as in adults, has proven to be successful and relatively well-tolerated. However, there is emerging data suggesting that long-term therapy causes side-effects that are specific to the pediatric setting. Specifically, evidence suggests that the use of imatinib and related tyrosine kinase inhibitors in children has effects on growth. This article will review available data from recent studies suggesting that these drugs may cause growth deceleration in prepubescent patients, leading to lasting effects on ultimate adult height. The putative mechanisms responsible for these effects on growth, including altered bone metabolism or growth hormone levels and direct effects on the growth plate, will be discussed. In addition, the implications of these observations on the use of tyrosine kinase inhibitors in the pediatric setting will be addressed.

Use of Imatinib in Children

Chronic myeloid leukemia (CML) is rarely seen in children, accounting for less than 3% of all childhood leukemias (Castro-Malaspina *et al.*, 1983, Kaatsch, 2010). Evidence suggests that the molecular and clinical features of the disease, and response to therapy, appear to be very similar in adults and children. Imatinib is the standard therapy for chronic phase Philadelphia chromosome-positive (Ph+) CML in adults and has proven to be similarly effective in children, with response rates that are similar to those seen in adults. The majority of children with chronic phase Ph+ CML receiving imatinib upfront achieve a complete cytogenetic response within the first year (Millot *et al.*, 2011, Champagne *et al.*, 2011). Following 12 months of treatment, 61% of pediatric Ph+ CML patients achieve a complete cytogenetic response and 31% achieve a major molecular response (Millot *et al.*, 2011). The estimated 3-year overall survival is 92% (Champagne *et al.*, 2011). In general, the side effects of imatinib in pediatric patients are similar to that found in adults, with a low incidence of grade 3/4 adverse reactions. However, unlike their adult counterparts, pediatric patients report a lower frequency of musculoskeletal pain and peripheral edema (Millot *et al.*, 2011, Champagne *et al.*, 2011).

Imatinib has been approved for use in pediatric chronic phase Ph+ CML upfront or when disease recurrence is evident following allogeneic stem cell transplantation, or when pediatric patients exhibit resistance or intolerance to interferon-α therapy. Consensus recommendations support the use of imatinib upfront in pediatric patients with chronic phase Ph+ CML. Previous recommendations suggested limiting exposure to imatinib therapy to up to 2 years even if an optimal response is achieved (Suttorp, 2008). However, most recent recommendations suggest that pediatric patients remain on imatinib indefinitely in cases of optimal response (Andolina *et al.*, 2012). In cases of suboptimal response to imatinib, recommendations suggest proceeding to transplant with the best identified hematopoietic stem cell donor (Andolina *et al.*, 2012) or, if an HLA-matched donor is not available, proceeding to the second generation tyrosine kinase inhibitor, dasatinib (Suttorp and Millot, 2010). For Ph+ CML in acute or blast phase, recommendations suggest commencing imatinib or dasatinib treatment and then proceeding to stem cell transplant from the best available donor once a hematologic or better cytogenetic response has been achieved (Suttorp and Millot, 2010, Andolina *et al.*, 2012).

Clinical Evidence for Growth Effects

While short-term imatinib therapy has been successful and well-tolerated in children with chronic-phase Ph+ CML (Giona *et al.*, 2008, Suttorp *et al.*, 2009, Millot *et al.*, 2011, Champagne *et al.*, 2011), there is emerging data suggesting that long-term therapy may result in side-effects that are specific to the pediatric setting. Specifically, impairment of linear growth is emerging as a commonly-observed complication of imatinib therapy in prepubescent patients.

Four case reports have noted growth retardation coinciding with the start of imatinib therapy in pre-pubescent CML cases (Mariani *et al.*, 2008, Kimoto *et al.*, 2009, Schmid *et al.*, 2009, Hobernicht *et al.*, 2011). Mariani *et al.* described an 11-year-old boy who experienced a dramatic reduction in growth rate from 4.3 cm/year to 1.5 cm/year after commencing imatinib therapy (Mariani *et al.*, 2008). While normal growth recommenced at the onset of puberty, 2 years after imatinib treatment began, the correlation of the onset of growth retardation with the onset of imatinib therapy suggested a causative link. A second report described a 6-year-old female whose growth velocity decreased after beginning imatinib therapy for CML (Kimoto *et al.*, 2009). During 4 years of imatinib therapy, the patient's height increased only marginally, from 114 cm to 121 cm, with a corresponding decrease in height standard deviation score (SDS) from -0.7 to -2.7. Furthermore, when imatinib therapy ceased, the patient's growth rate rapidly increased. Schmid *et al.* recently reported decreased growth in a female CML patient who commenced treatment with imatinib at age 5.5 years. This patient's height was in the 74th percentile at diagnosis; however, it fell to the 9th percentile after 3 years of imatinib treatment (Schmid *et al.*, 2009). Finally, Hobernicht *et al.* reported on a 7-year-old girl who experienced growth deceleration whilst undergoing imatinib treatment for CML (Hobernicht *et al.*, 2011). The patient's height percentile decreased from the 75th percentile when diagnosed with CML to the 25th percentile after 5 years of imatinib therapy.

Additionally, a French phase IV trial has reported decreased growth in a cohort of 22 children and adolescents (age: 10 months – 17 years) receiving imatinib therapy for chronic phase CML (Millot *et al.*, 2009). Growth rate in this group was significantly lower following imatinib treatment, with a significant decrease in height SDS (median: -0.37; range: -1.09 – +0.14) after 12 months of treatment, compared with baseline (Millot *et al.*, 2009).

In one of the most long-term studies to date, Shima *et al.* followed 48 chronic phase CML children for a median of 34 months (range: 10 – 88 months) (Shima *et al.*, 2011). In this study, 73% of patients had a decrease in growth rate, with a median maximal yearly fall in height SDS of -0.61 over the period of monitoring. Interestingly, growth tended to recover after reaching puberty. Fifty percent (4/8) of patients followed into the pubertal age range displayed catch up growth. Additionally, when the group was divided into patients who commenced treatment prior to puberty (n = 27) and those who started treatment when in puberty (n = 21), height SDS began to decline within the first year of treatment in prepubertal patients, while in pubertal patients height remained steady throughout treatment.

A similar observation was noted in a retrospective analysis of growth in 20 pediatric patients (median age: 10 years, range: 2 – 13) receiving imatinib therapy for a mean duration of 61 months (range: 31 – 83) (Bansal *et al.*, 2012). In this study, a significant reduction in height SDS was observed in prepubescent patients (n = 13; P = 0.003), while no change in height SDS was detectable in pubescent patients (n = 7; P = 0.448), after 5 years of treatment.

Furthermore, a retrospective single center analysis of growth in 7 pediatric patients treated with imatinib showed that 5/7 patients displayed a decrease in height SDS following imatinib treatment, when compared with prior to therapy (Rastogi *et al.*, 2012). Notably, while 4 of these patients showed improved growth velocity at the onset of puberty, 3 patients failed to achieve their predicted adult height, as based on mid-parental target height.

While these studies suggest that imatinib therapy in pre-pubertal individuals may retard growth, there are currently few reports suggesting potential mechanisms for the altered growth in imatinib-treated pediatric patients. Below we discuss several potential mechanisms for the observed effects of imatinib on growth, including aberrant bone formation and resorption, accelerated growth plate closure, and effects on growth hormone (GH).

Mechanism

Effects of Imatinib on Skeletal Metabolism

A number of studies have documented that imatinib has unanticipated off target effects on bone remodeling in adults, resulting in regional changes in bone mineral density (BMD) and sustained decreases in serum phosphate (hyperphosphatemia) and elevated parathyroid hormone levels (hyperparathyroidism). Retrospective and longitudinal studies from our group have shown that, relative to baseline, CML patients receiving imatinib exhibit significantly increased trabecular bone volume in iliac crest bone biopsies (Fitter *et al.*, 2008, Vandyke et al., 2013). Using dual-energy X-ray absorptiometry (DXA), a number of studies have demonstrated that regional BMD measurements at the lumbar spine (Jönsson *et al.*, 2008, O'Sullivan *et al.*, 2009), total hip (Jönsson *et al.*, 2008) and distal radius (Vandyke et al., 2013) are increased in imatinib-treated patients. Additionally, peripheral quantitative computed tomography (pQCT) analysis revealed that the radial and tibial cortical BMD, but not trabecular BMD, was significantly higher in the imatinib-treated group when compared with a healthy control group (Jönsson *et al.*, 2008). In contrast, a recent study from our group shows that femoral neck BMD is significantly decreased as early as 6 months following commencement of imatinib therapy (Vandyke et al., 2013). Collectively, these data strongly suggest that imatinib alters bone remodeling in adult patients.

While the mechanism(s) remain to be fully elucidated, these changes primarily appear to relate to a decrease in osteoclastic bone resorption that is not corrected by a concomitant decrease in bone formation by osteoblasts. Our group were the first to identify that imatinib has strong inhibitory effects on osteoclast formation/survival and activity *in vitro* through inhibition of the macrophage colony stimulating factor (M-CSF) receptor Fms and, potentially, Kit, carbonic anhydrase II (CAII) and platelet-derived growth factor receptor (PDGFR)-α and -β (Dewar *et al.*, 2006, Ando *et al.*, 2006, El Hajj Dib *et al.*, 2006, O'Sullivan *et al.*, 2007, Vandyke *et al.*, 2010b). Furthermore, decreased serum markers of osteoclast activity have consistently been observed in CML and GIST patients treated with imatinib. Berman *et al.* identified that serum levels of the osteoclast marker N-telopeptide of collagen crosslinks were decreased in imatinib-treated CML and GIST patients, relative to healthy controls (Berman *et al.*, 2006). Longitudinal studies subsequently confirmed that serum osteoclast markers are decreased following imatinib therapy (O'Sullivan *et al.*, 2009, Vandyke et al., 2013). Furthermore, we have recently demonstrated that these decreases in serum osteoclast markers are associated with a marked decrease in osteoclast numbers in iliac crest trephine biopsies in imatinib-treated CML patients, when compared with prior to treatment (Vandyke et al., 2013). Taken together, these results strongly suggest that imatinib is a direct inhibitor of osteoclast survival, differentiation and activity both *in vitro* and in patients.

Furthermore, there is considerable evidence that imatinib decreases osteoblast progenitor proliferation while increasing osteoblast differentiation and mineralized matrix production *in vitro*, at least in part through inhibition of PDGFR (Fierro *et al.*, 2007, O'Sullivan *et al.*, 2007, Fitter *et al.*, 2008, Wihlidal *et al.*, 2008, Tibullo *et al.*, 2009, Jönsson *et al.*, 2011). However, the implications for these effects in patients are less clear, with conflicting data regarding the effects of imatinib on serum markers of osteoblast activity in patients. In cross-sectional studies, serum osteocalcin levels have been shown to be significantly decreased in imatinib-treated CML and GIST patients, relative to healthy controls, while serum bone-specific alkaline phosphatase levels were similar between these groups (Berman *et al.*, 2006, Jönsson *et al.*, 2008). In contrast, some longitudinal studies have observed increases in serum osteocalcin and P1NP levels at the early stages of imatinib therapy, which either return to baseline levels by 18 months (O'Sullivan *et al.*, 2009) or are sustained until at least 24 months of treatment (Tibullo *et al.*, 2009). Importantly, a longitudinal histological study of 11 Ph+

CML patients has demonstrated no changes in osteoblast numbers or osteoid parameters in iliac crest biopsies (Vandyke et al., 2013). Similarly, no significant changes in serum osteocalcin and P1NP levels were observed in CML patients over 24 months of imatinib treatment (Vandyke et al., 2013). When taken together, these data suggest that imatinib therapy dysregulates bone remodeling in adult patients by mediating a decrease in osteoclast numbers and activity which is not counteracted by a concomitant decrease in osteoblast activity.

While the effects of imatinib on the mature adult skeleton are well characterized, there is a paucity of data regarding the effects of imatinib on bone metabolism in pediatric patients, where the skeleton is actively modeling, rather than remodeling. One case report has examined markers of bone biochemistry in a female CML patient after 17 to 34 months of imatinib therapy (age: 7 – 8.5 years) (Schmid *et al.*, 2009). This patient was found to have reduced serum P1NP levels, increased serum osteocalcin, and normal levels of bone-specific alkaline phosphatase, compared with the age-matched normal range. The patient also exhibited increased urinary excretion of the osteoclast markers pyridinoline (PYR) and desoxypyridinoline (DPYR), suggesting an increase in osteoclast activity. Additionally, one cross-sectional study has examined serum markers of osteoclast and osteoblast activity in 57 pediatric patients who were receiving imatinib treatment (Suttorp and Millot, 2010). In contrast to the potent anti-osteoclastic effects of imatinib seen in adult cohort, urinary levels of the osteoclast marker deoxypyrodinoline were in the normal range in the vast majority of imatinib-treated pediatric patients. However, there was an inverse correlation with length of treatment, suggesting that osteoclast activity may decrease with prolonged treatment in pediatric patients. In contrast, serum levels of the osteoblast marker osteocalcin were elevated above the normal range in 33/57 (58%) of imatinib-treated pediatric patients. Similarly, there was a statistically significant trend towards decreasing osteocalcin levels with increasing duration of treatment, although levels were still generally elevated above the age and sex-adjusted normal range after 2 years of treatment. As neither of these studies compared their results with base-line, pre-treatment assessments, it is difficult to determine the overall effects of imatinib on bone remodeling in pediatric patients. Longitudinal studies are warranted to assess the effects of imatinib on markers of bone remodeling in children, to investigate whether imatinib causes effects on the skeleton which could account for the associated effects on growth.

Effects of Imatinib on the Growth Plate

Longitudinal bone growth is tightly regulated through the coordinated proliferation, differentiation and activity of epiphyseal growth plate chondrocytes (reviewed by (Villemure and Stokes, 2009)). In normal bone, the rate of chondrocyte proliferation and the size of the resultant hypertrophic chondrocytes are the primary determinants of the rate of longitudinal bone growth (Hunziker and Schenk, 1989, Wilsman *et al.*, 1996, Ballock and O'Keefe, 2003). Chondrocyte proliferation and maturation is tightly-regulated by autocrine and paracrine signalling, the disruption of which can cause aberrant bone growth, resulting in a number of human growth disorders (Shiang *et al.*, 1994, Bellus *et al.*, 1995, Tavormina *et al.*, 1995, Woods and Savage, 1996). Studies emerging from our laboratory suggest that imatinib treatment causes premature growth plate closure *in vivo*, suggesting a potential mechanism for the observed growth delay in imatinib-treated pre-pubescent patients (Vandyke *et al.*, 2009b). In these studies, we showed that imatinib treatment of normal 9-month-old Sprague-Dawley rats significantly decreased growth plate thickness, resulting in complete fusion of the growth plate after 3 months of treatment. In addition, a study by Nurmio and colleagues demonstrated that short-term imatinib treatment of young rats resulted in a rapid decrease in growth plate thickness and a sustained decrease in size (Nurmio *et al.*, 2011). This study demonstrated that 3-day treatment of 5-day-old Sprague Dawley rats resulted in a small but sustained delay in growth, such that 10 weeks after withdrawal of treatment imatinib-treated animals were approximately 10% smaller that the control group. Furthermore, treatment with imatinib resulted in a significant thinning of the proximal tibial growth plates, corresponding to a reduction in proliferating and hypertrophic zone thickness. These effects on the growth plate may be due to direct effects on chondrocyte proliferation and differentiation, as imatinib inhibits cell proliferation and extracellular matrix synthesis in cultures of chondrocyte-like cells *in vitro*, at least in part through inhibition of PDGFR-β signalling (Vandyke *et al.*, 2009b). However, given the broad target specificities of imatinib, other tyrosine kinases, such as discoidin domain receptor 2 (DDR2) (Bantscheff *et al.*, 2007, Labrador *et al.*, 2001, Leitinger and Kwan, 2006), may also play a role in the effects of imatinib on chondrogenesis.

Growth plate thickness is determined by rate of chondrocyte proliferation and hypertrophy and by the rate of replacement of the cartilagenous matrix with mature bone (Parfitt, 2002). Therefore, stimulation of osteoblast activity by imatinib (Fierro *et al.*, 2007, O'Sullivan *et al.*, 2007, Fitter *et al.*, 2008, Wihlidal *et al.*, 2008, Tibullo *et al.*, 2009, Jönsson *et al.*, 2011) may have additional effects on growth plate thickness by accelerating growth plate mineralization. Supporting this, in the study by Nurmio *et al.*, the decrease in growth plate thickness in imatinib-treated rats was associated with a dramatic decrease in osteoclast numbers and a slight increase in osteoblast numbers at the osteochondral junction, leading to a hypothetical increase in bone formation. However, the authors failed to provide an explanation for the decreased trabecular BMD which was also observed at this site.

Notably, growth plate closure in healthy vertebrates is a marker of growth cessation, rather than a cause of it (Parfitt, 2002). It is not clear from existing studies whether the rapid acceleration of growth plate closure observed in rats is merely associated with a growth inhibitory effect of imatinib therapy, or is a mechanism by which imatinib therapy causes decreased growth. In 7 of the reported cases of delayed growth in imatinib-treated pre-pubescent patients, bone age (based on X-rays of the wrist or hand) was delayed (Kimoto *et al.*, 2009, Schmid *et al.*, 2009, Rastogi *et al.*, 2012) or normal (Mariani *et al.*, 2008), indicating that premature growth plate closure at these sites was not evident. However, this does not rule out the possibility that the growth plates were affected at other sites. Moreover, the resumption of growth in the majority of patients at the onset of puberty (Mariani *et al.*, 2008, Shima *et al.*, 2011, Bansal *et al.*, 2012, Rastogi *et al.*, 2012) or following cessation of treatment (Kimoto *et al.*, 2009) also suggests that complete growth plate closure is unlikely to be occurring in imatinib-treated children. In any case, the dramatic effect of imatinib on growth plate closure in rats suggests that growth plate morphology should be monitored in juvenile patients undergoing imatinib therapy, and should be investigated as a potential mechanism for inhibited growth in pre-pubescent patients receiving imatinib. While the inhibition of chondrocyte proliferation and activity may have detrimental effects on growth, the potential that imatinib causes growth retardation through other mechanisms such as effect on GH, must also be considered.

Growth Hormone Deficiency

Longitudinal bone growth in childhood is primarily dependent upon the release and response to GH. GH acts directly at the growth plate to stimulate chrondrocyte proliferation, and also has indirect effects through the induction of insulin-like growth factor 1 (IGF-1) production by the liver and locally at the growth plate, which further stimulates longitudinal bone growth.

Several studies have identified potential GH deficiency in some, but not all, pediatric patients who exhibit growth retardation whilst undergoing imatinib therapy. In a group of 4 pediatric patients receiving imatinib, IGF-1 and IGF-binding protein-3 (IGFBP-3) were within the normal range in all patients during treatment, suggesting a normal GH response (Rastogi *et al.*, 2012). Another child was similarly reported to have normal GH and IGF-1 levels during imatinib treatment (Mariani *et al.*, 2008). In contrast, one child was reported to have low serum IGF-1 levels, but a normal IGF-1 release in response to GH stimulation, indicating a potential defect in GH secretion (Hobernicht *et al.*, 2011). A further child was found to have borderline low IGF-1 during imatinib therapy, which may indicate a partial GH deficiency (Schmid *et al.*, 2009). In a cohort of 17 adult imatinib-treated CML patients, 25 – 75% of patients had GH deficiency, as defined by low serum levels of IGF-1 and IGFBP-3 and decreased GH release in response to glucagon or L-DOPA stimulation (Kebapcilar *et al.*, 2009). However, as an imatinib-naïve CML cohort was not examined in any of these studies, it is unclear whether any observed deficiency was due to treatment or resulted from illness. Nonetheless, the possibility that GH deficiency may contribute to the decreased growth in some imatinib-treated patients should be further investigated.

Potential Effects of the Second Generation TKI Dasatinib on Growth

In response to the success of dasatinib as a frontline treatment for adult patients (Kantarjian *et al.*, 2010), dasatinib is now being considered as a treatment for Ph+ chronic phase CML in children and adolescents who are resistant or intolerant to imatinib (Zwaan *et al.*, 2008, Aplenc *et al.*, 2008, Suttorp and Millot, 2010) or as an alternate upfront treatment to imatinib (Andolina *et al.*, 2012). Furthermore, dasatinib is also recommended as an upfront treatment for pediatric Ph+ CML in acute or blast phase (Andolina *et al.*, 2012). While dasatinib is not yet approved for these applications, emerging clinical trials have shown promising results for dasatinib in the pediatric setting.

The Innovative Therapies for Children with Cancer (ITCC) Consortium has conducted a phase I trial of dasatinib in children with relapsed or refractory Ph+ leukemias (Zwaan *et al.*, 2010). In patients with imatinib-resistant or intolerant chronic phase Ph+ CML, treatment responses were excellent, with complete hematologic responses observed in 16/17 (94%) patients, complete cytogenetic response in 14/17 (82%) patients, and complete molecular response in 4/17 (24%) patients after a median of 11.3 months of treatment (range: 2.3 – 47.9) (Zwaan *et al.*, 2010). A phase I Children's Oncology Group trial of dasatinib in children with refractory solid tumours or leukemias reported a partial or better cytogenetic response in 6/8 patients with chronic phase Ph+ CML, with 3 patients achieving a complete cytogenetic response (Aplenc *et al.*, 2011). These preliminary results suggest that dasatinib may be a highly effective treatment for children with imatinib resistant or intolerant CML.

Dasatinib, like imatinib, inhibits the activity of Abl, Fms, and the PDGF family members Kit and PDGFR-α and -β (Lombardo *et al.*, 2004, Melnick *et al.*, 2006, Shah *et al.*, 2004, O'Hare *et al.*, 2005, Vandyke *et al.*, 2009a, Brownlow *et al.*, 2009). Additionally, dasatinib is a potent inhibitor of the Src-family kinases (Src, Lck, Hck, Yes, Fgr, Lyn and Fyn) (Lombardo *et al.*, 2004, Bantscheff *et al.*, 2007). Given the overlapping target specificities of imatinib and dasatinib, it is likely that dasatinib may have similar growth effects as imatinib.

One case report has suggested that dasatinib, like imatinib, may have negative effects on growth in prepubescent patients (Hobernicht *et al.*, 2011). In this report, a girl exhibiting significant growth retardation and GH deficiency whilst undergoing imatinib therapy was subsequently switched to treatment with dasatinib. Upon transferring to dasatinib, there was no improvement in longitudinal growth. Furthermore, the patient showed defective GH release in response to stimulus tests with clonidine or arginine, suggesting continuing GH deficiency. This study suggests that dasatinib may cause growth inhibition in pediatric patients, although further studies are required to confirm this association.

Studies have demonstrated that dasatinib, like imatinib, can cause decreased growth plate thickness in normal Sprague-Dawley rats (Vandyke *et al.*, 2011). This was found to be, in part, associated with a decrease in chondrocyte proliferation and activity, through inhibition of PDGFR (Vandyke *et al.*, 2011). Furthermore, inhibition of Src-family kinases by dasatinib may also contribute to decreased chondrocyte proliferation (Bursell *et al.*, 2007, Pala *et al.*, 2008). In addition to inhibiting chondrocyte proliferation and activity, dasatinib can affect osteoblast activity, inhibiting stromal cell proliferation while, under at least some conditions, promoting osteoblast activity (Vandyke *et al.*, 2010a, Lee *et al.*, 2010, Id Boufker *et al.*, 2010, Vandyke *et al.*, 2011, Garcia-Gomez *et al.*, 2012). Furthermore, dasatinib is a potent inhibitor of osteoclastogenesis which, at clinically-relevant concentrations, inhibits the formation and activity of osteoclasts from human peripheral blood mononuclear cells and primary mouse and rat bone marrow cells *in vitro* (Vandyke *et al.*, 2009a, Brownlow *et al.*, 2009, Garcia-Gomez *et al.*, 2012, Vandyke *et al.*, 2010a). In normal skeletally-mature rats, dasatinib treatment resulted in increased trabecular BMD through an inhibition of osteoclast formation or survival, which was not balanced by a decrease in osteoblast activity (Vandyke *et al.*, 2010a). It remains to be determined what effect this may have on bone remodeling in patients undergoing dasatinib treatment.

Implications

As highlighted by this review, there is a need for prospective studies elucidating the effects of imatinib and dasatinib therapy on growth, the growth plate, skeletal metabolism and GH levels in pediatric CML patients. We suggest that growth plate changes and skeletal metabolism should be monitored in pediatric patients that are undergoing treatment with tyrosine kinase inhibitors. Furthermore, GH deficiency should be considered as a potential cause of delayed growth in imatinib-treated pediatric patients.

Current consensus recommendations agree that imatinib, or perhaps dasatinib, is the best option upfront for pediatric CML patients. However, the relative benefit of long-term imatinib and dasatinib as a frontline treatment for diseases affecting children and adolescents needs to be re-evaluated, taking into account the potential effects of imatinib and dasatinib on growth. The consequences of inhibited growth in pediatric patients may be marked, and, although evidence suggests that most, if not all, patients will resume growth upon the onset of puberty, it is likely that they will never reach their genetic target height. Considering that the current paradigm suggests that patients may remain on imatinib indefinitely, the relative advantages of this long term treatment, versus the risks associated with the curative option of hematopoietic stem cell transplant, should be considered in the light of these potential effects of imatinib on growth. However, ultimately the potential side effect of imatinib on growth is not likely to direct therapeutic options in most cases, as the alternate treatment strategy, hematopoietic stem cell transplant, is itself associated with significant treatment-related mortality and long-term morbidities including graft versus host disease, infertility, endocrine deficiencies and impaired growth (Sanders, 2002, Sanders *et al.*, 2005, Couto-Silva *et al.*, 2006, Cohen *et al.*, 2008, Tichelli *et al.*, 2009).

References

[1] Ando, W., Hashimoto, J., Nampei, A., Tsuboi, H., Tateishi, K., Ono, T., Nakamura, N., Ochi, T. & Yoshikawa, H. 2006. Imatinib Mesylate Inhibits Osteoclastogenesis And Joint Destruction In Rats With Collagen-Induced Arthritis (Cia). *J Bone Miner Metab,* 24, 274-82.

[2] Andolina, J. R., Neudorf, S. M. & Corey, S. J. 2012. How I Treat Childhood Cml. *Blood,* 119, 1821-30.

[3] Aplenc, R., Blaney, S. M., Strauss, L. C., Balis, F. M., Shusterman, S., Ingle, A. M., Agrawal, S., Sun, J., Wright, J. J. & Adamson, P. C. 2011. Pediatric Phase I Trial And Pharmacokinetic Study Of Dasatinib: A Report From The Children's Oncology Group Phase I Consortium. *Journal Of Clinical Oncology,* 29, 839-44.

[4] Aplenc, R., Strauss, L. C., Shusterman, S., Ingle, A. M., Agrawal, S., Sun, J., Wright, J. J., Blaney, S. M. & P.C., A. 2008. Pediatric Phase I Trial And Pharmacokinetic (Pk) Study Of Dasatinib: A Report From The Children's Oncology Group Phase I Consortium. *Journal Of Clinical Oncology,* 26, 3591.

[5] Ballock, R. T. & O'keefe, R. J. 2003. The Biology Of The Growth Plate. *J Bone Joint Surg Am,* 85-A, 715-26.

[6] Bansal, D., Shava, U., Varma, N., Trehan, A. & Marwaha, R. K. 2012. Imatinib Has Adverse Effect On Growth In Children With Chronic Myeloid Leukemia. *Pediatric Blood & Cancer,* 59, 481-4.

[7] Bantscheff, M., Eberhard, D., Abraham, Y., Bastuck, S., Boesche, M., Hobson, S., Mathieson, T., Perrin, J., Raida, M., Rau, C., Reader, V., Sweetman, G., Bauer, A., Bouwmeester, T., Hopf, C., Kruse, U., Neubauer, G., Ramsden, N., Rick, J., Kuster, B. & Drewes, G. 2007. Quantitative Chemical Proteomics Reveals Mechanisms Of Action Of Clinical Abl Kinase Inhibitors. *Nat Biotechnol,* 25, 1035-44.

[8] Bellus, G. A., Hefferon, T. W., Ortiz De Luna, R. I., Hecht, J. T., Horton, W. A., Machado, M., Kaitila, I., Mcintosh, I. & Francomano, C. A. 1995. Achondroplasia Is Defined By Recurrent G380r Mutations Of Fgfr3. *Am J Hum Genet,* 56, 368-73.

[9] Berman, E., Nicolaides, M., Maki, R. G., Fleisher, M., Chanel, S., Scheu, K., Wilson, B. A., Heller, G. & Sauter, N. P. 2006. Altered Bone And Mineral Metabolism In Patients Receiving Imatinib Mesylate. *N Engl J Med,* 354, 2006-13.

[10] Brownlow, N., Mol, C., Hayford, C., Ghaem-Maghami, S. & Dibb, N. J. 2009. Dasatinib Is A Potent Inhibitor Of Tumour-Associated Macrophages, Osteoclasts And The Fms Receptor. *Leukemia,* 23, 590-4.

[11] Bursell, L., Woods, A., James, C. G., Pala, D., Leask, A. & Beier, F. 2007. Src Kinase Inhibition Promotes The Chondrocyte Phenotype. *Arthritis Res Ther,* 9, R105.

[12] Castro-Malaspina, H., Schaison, G., Briere, J., Passe, S., Pasquier, A., Tanzer, J., Jacquillat, C. & Bernard, J. 1983. Philadelphia Chromosome-Positive Chronic Myelocytic Leukemia In Children. Survival And Prognostic Factors. *Cancer,* 52, 721-7.

[13] Champagne, M. A., Fu, C. H., Chang, M., Chen, H., Gerbing, R. B., Alonzo, T. A., Cooley, L. D., Heerema, N. A., Oehler, V., Wood, C., French, M. E., Arceci, R. J., Smith, F. O. & Bernstein, M. L. 2011. Higher Dose Imatinib For Children With De Novo Chronic Phase Chronic Myelogenous Leukemia: A Report From The Children's Oncology Group. *Pediatric Blood & Cancer,* 57, 56-62.

[14] Cohen, A., Bekassy, A. N., Gaiero, A., Faraci, M., Zecca, S., Tichelli, A. & Dini, G. 2008. Endocrinological Late Complications After Hematopoietic Sct In Children. *Bone Marrow Transplantation,* 41 Suppl 2, S43-8.

[15] Couto-Silva, A. C., Trivin, C., Esperou, H., Michon, J., Baruchel, A., Lemaire, P. & Brauner, R. 2006. Final Height And Gonad Function After Total Body Irradiation During Childhood. *Bone Marrow Transplantation,* 38, 427-32.

[16] Dewar, A. L., Farrugia, A. N., Condina, M. R., Bik To, L., Hughes, T. P., Vernon-Roberts, B. & Zannettino, A. C. W. 2006. Imatinib As A Potential Antiresorptive Therapy For Bone Disease. *Blood,* 107, 4334-7.

[17] El Hajj Dib, I., Gallet, M., Mentaverri, R., Sevenet, N., Brazier, M. & Kamel, S. 2006. Imatinib Mesylate (Gleevec) Enhances Mature Osteoclast Apoptosis And Suppresses Osteoclast Bone Resorbing Activity. *Eur J Pharmacol,* 551, 27-33.

[18] Fierro, F., Illmer, T., Jing, D., Schleyer, E., Ehninger, G., Boxberger, S. & Bornhäuser, M. 2007. Inhibition Of Platelet-Derived Growth Factor Receptor□ By Imatinib Mesylate Suppresses Proliferation And Alters Differentiation Of Human Mesenchymal Stem Cells *In Vitro*. *Cell Prolif,* 40, 355-66.

[19] Fitter, S., Dewar, A. L., Kostakis, P., To, L. B., Hughes, T. P., Roberts, M. M., Lynch, K., Vernon-Roberts, B. & Zannettino, A. C. W. 2008. Long-Term Imatinib Therapy Promotes Bone Formation In Cml Patients. *Blood,* 111, 2538-47.

[20] Garcia-Gomez, A., Ocio, E. M., Crusoe, E., Santamaria, C., Hernandez-Campo, P., Blanco, J. F., Sanchez-Guijo, F. M., Hernandez-Iglesias, T., Brinon, J. G., Fisac-Herrero, R. M., Lee, F. Y., Pandiella, A., San Miguel, J. F. & Garayoa, M. 2012. Dasatinib As A Bone-Modifying Agent: Anabolic And Anti-Resorptive Effects. *Plos One,* 7, E34914.

[21] Giona, F., Putti, M. C., Moleti, M. L., Nanni, M., Testi, A. M., Varotto, S., Gottardi, E. M., De Vellis, A., Nunes, V., Diverio, D., Leszl, A., Saglio, G. & Foà, R. 2008. Imatinib Mesylate Induces High Complete Cytogenetic And Molecular Response Rates In Children And Adolescents With Philadelphia Chromosome-Positive (Ph+) Chronic Myelogenous Leukemia (Cml) In Chronic Phase (Cp) [Abstract]. *Blood,* 122, 4273.

[22] Obernicht, S. L., Schweiger, B., Zeitler, P., Wang, M. & Hunger, S. P. 2011. Acquired Growth Hormone Deficiency In A Girl With Chronic Myelogenous Leukemia Treated With Tyrosine Kinase Inhibitor Therapy. *Pediatric Blood & Cancer,* 56, 671-3.

[23] Hunziker, E. B. & Schenk, R. K. 1989. Physiological Mechanisms Adopted By Chondrocytes In Regulating Longitudinal Bone Growth In Rats. *J Physiol,* 414, 55-71.

[24] Id Boufker, H., Lagneaux, L., Najar, M., Piccart, M., Ghanem, G., Body, J. J. & Journé, F. 2010. The Src Inhibitor Dasatinib Accelerates The Differentiation Of Human Bone Marrow-Derived Mesenchymal Stromal Cells Into Osteoblasts. *Bmc Cancer,* 10, 298.

[25] Jönsson, S., Hjorth-Hansen, H., Olsson, B., Wadenvik, H., Sundan, A. & Standal, T. 2011. Imatinib Inhibits Proliferation Of Human Mesenchymal Stem Cells And Promotes Early But Not Late Osteoblast Differentiation *In Vitro. J Bone Miner Metab.*

[26] Jönsson, S., Olsson, B., Ohlsson, C., Lorentzon, M., Mellström, D. & Wadenvik, H. 2008. Increased Cortical Bone Mineralization In Imatinib Treated Patients With Chronic Myelogenous Leukemia. *Hematologica,* 93, 1101-3.

[27] Kaatsch, P. 2010. Epidemiology Of Childhood Cancer. *Cancer Treat Rev,* 36, 277-85.

[28] Kantarjian, H., Shah, N. P., Hochhaus, A., Cortes, J., Shah, S., Ayala, M., Moiraghi, B., Shen, Z., Mayer, J., Pasquini, R., Nakamae, H., Huguet, F., Boque, C., Chuah, C., Bleickardt, E., Bradley-Garelik, M. B., Zhu, C., Szatrowski, T., Shapiro, D. & Baccarani, M. 2010. Dasatinib Versus Imatinib In Newly Diagnosed Chronic-Phase Chronic Myeloid Leukemia. *N Engl J Med,* 362, 2260-70.

[29] Kebapcilar, L., Bilgir, O., Alacacioglu, I., Payzin, B., Bilgir, F., Oner, P., Sari, I., Calan, M. & Binicier, O. 2009. Does Imatinib Mesylate Therapy Cause Growth Hormone Deficiency? *Med Princ Pract,* 18, 360-3.

[30] Kimoto, T., Inoue, M. & Kawa, K. 2009. Growth Deceleration In A Girl Treated With Imatinib. *Int J Hematol,* 89, 251-2.

[31] Labrador, J. P., Azcoitia, V., Tuckermann, J., Lin, C., Olaso, E., Manes, S., Bruckner, K., Goergen, J. L., Lemke, G., Yancopoulos, G., Angel, P., Martinez, C. & Klein, R. 2001. The Collagen Receptor Ddr2 Regulates Proliferation And Its Elimination Leads To Dwarfism. *Embo Rep,* 2, 446-52.

[32] Lee, Y. C., Huang, C. F., Murshed, M., Chu, K., Araujo, J. C., Ye, X., Decrombrugghe, B., Yu-Lee, L. Y., Gallick, G. E. & Lin, S. H. 2010. Src Family Kinase/Abl Inhibitor Dasatinib Suppresses Proliferation And Enhances Differentiation Of Osteoblasts. *Oncogene,* Prepublished On March 15, 2010 As Doi 10.1038/Onc.2010.73.

[33] Leitinger, B. & Kwan, A. P. 2006. The Discoidin Domain Receptor Ddr2 Is A Receptor For Type X Collagen. *Matrix Biol,* 25, 355-64.

[34] Lombardo, L. J., Lee, F. Y., Chen, P., Norris, D., Barrish, J. C., Behnia, K., Castaneda, S., Cornelius, L. A., Das, J., Doweyko, A. M., Fairchild, C., Hunt, J. T., Inigo, I., Johnston, K., Kamath, A., Kan, D., Klei, H., Marathe, P., Pang, S., Peterson, R., Pitt, S., Schieven, G. L., Schmidt, R. J., Tokarski, J., Wen, M.-L., Wityak, J. & Borzilleri, R. M. 2004. Discovery Of N-(2-Chloro-6-Methyl- Phenyl)-2-(6-(4-(2-Hydroxyethyl)-Piperazin-1-Yl)-2-Methylpyrimidin-4- Ylamino)Thiazole-5-Carboxamide (Bms-354825), A Dual Src/Abl Kinase Inhibitor With Potent Antitumor Activity In Preclinical Assays. *J Med Chem,* 47, 6658-61.

[35] Mariani, S., Giona, F., Basciani, S., Brama, M. & Gnessi, L. 2008. Low Bone Density And Decreased Inhibin-B/Fsh Ratio In A Boy Treated With Imatinib During Puberty. *Lancet,* 372, 111-2.

[36] Melnick, J. S., Janes, J., Kim, S., Chang, J. Y., Sipes, D. G., Gunderson, D., Jarnes, L., Matzen, J. T., Garcia, M. E., Hood, T. L., Beigi, R., Xia, G., Harig, R. A., Asatryan, H., Yan, S. F., Zhou, Y., Gu, X.-J., Saadat, A., Zhou, V., King, F. J., Shaw, C. M., Su, A. I., Downs, R., Gray, N. S., Schultz, P. G., Warmuth, M. & Caldwell, J. S. 2006. An Efficient Rapid System For Profiling The Cellular Activities Of Molecular Libraries. *Proc Natl Acad Sci U S A,* 103**,** 3153-8.

[37] Millot, F., Baruchel, A., Guilhot, J., Petit, A., Leblanc, T., Bertrand, Y., Mazingue, F., Lutz, P., Verite, C., Berthou, C., Galambrun, C., Bernard, F., Yacouben, K., Bordigoni, P., Edan, C., Reguerre, Y., Couillault, G., Mechinaud, F., Cayuela, J. M. & Guilhot, F. 2011. Imatinib Is Effective In Children With Previously Untreated Chronic Myelogenous Leukemia In Early Chronic Phase: Results Of The French National Phase Iv Trial. *Journal Of Clinical Oncology,* 29**,** 2827-32.

[38] Millot, F., Baruchel, A., Guilhot, J., Petit, A., Leblanc, T., Bertrand, Y., Mazingue, F., Patrick, L., Vérité, C., Berthoux, C., Galambrun, C., Bernard, F., Yacouben, K., Bordigoni, P., Edan, C., Reguerre, Y., Couillaud, G., Cayuela, J.-M. & Guilhot, F. 2009. Imatinib Is Efficient But Has A Negative Impact On Growth In Children With Previously Untreated Chronic Myelogenous Leukaemia (Cml) In Early Chronic Phase (Cp): Results Of The French National Phase Iv Trial [Abstract]. *Blood,* 114**,** 863.

[39] Nurmio, M., Joki, H., Kallio, J., Maatta, J. A., Vaananen, H. K., Toppari, J., Jahnukainen, K. & Laitala-Leinonen, T. 2011. Receptor Tyrosine Kinase Inhibition Causes Simultaneous Bone Loss And Excess Bone Formation Within Growing Bone In Rats. *Toxicology And Applied Pharmacology,* 254**,** 267-79.

[40] O'hare, T., Walters, D. K., Stoffregen, E. P., Jia, T., Manley, P. W., Mestan, J., Cowan-Jacob, S. W., Lee, F. Y., Heinrich, M. C., Deininger, M. W. N. & Druker, B. J. 2005. *In Vitro* Activity Of Bcr-Abl Inhibitors Amn107 And Bms-354825 Against Clinically Relevant Imatinib-Resistant Abl Kinase Domain Mutants. *Cancer Res,* 65**,** 4500-5.

[41] O'sullivan, S., Horne, A., Wattie, D., Porteous, F., Callon, K., Gamble, G., Ebeling, P., Browett, P. & Grey, A. 2009. Decreased Bone Turnover Despite Persistent Secondary Hyperparathyroidism During Prolonged Treatment With Imatinib. *J Clin Endocrinol Metab,* 94**,** 1131-6.

[42] O'Sullivan, S., Naot, D., Callon, K., Porteous, F., Horne, A., Wattie, D., Watson, M., Cornish, J., Browett, P. & Grey, A. 2007. Imatinib Promotes Osteoblast Differentiation By Inhibiting Pdgfr Signaling And Inhibits Osteoclastogenesis By Both Direct And Stromal Cell-Dependent Mechanisms. *J Bone Miner Res,* 22**,** 1679-1689.

[43] Pala, D., Kapoor, M., Woods, A., Kennedy, L., Liu, S., Chen, S., Bursell, L., Lyons, K. M., Carter, D. E., Beier, F. & Leask, A. 2008. Focal Adhesion Kinase/Src Suppresses Early Chondrogenesis: Central Role Of Ccn2. *J Biol Chem,* 283**,** 9239-47.

[44] Parfitt, A. M. 2002. Misconceptions (1): Epiphyseal Fusion Causes Cessation Of Growth. *Bone,* 30**,** 337-9.

[45] Rastogi, M. V., Stork, L., Druker, B., Blasdel, C., Nguyen, T. & Boston, B. A. 2012. Imatinib Mesylate Causes Growth Deceleration In Pediatric Patients With Chronic Myelogenous Leukemia. *Pediatric Blood & Cancer.*

[46] Sanders, J. E. 2002. Chronic Graft-Versus-Host Disease And Late Effects After Hematopoietic Stem Cell Transplantation. *International Journal Of Hematology,* 76 Suppl 2**,** 15-28.

[47] Sanders, J. E., Guthrie, K. A., Hoffmeister, P. A., Woolfrey, A. E., Carpenter, P. A. & Appelbaum, F. R. 2005. Final Adult Height Of Patients Who Received Hematopoietic Cell Transplantation In Childhood. *Blood,* 105, 1348-54.

[48] Schmid, H., Jaeger, B. A., Lohse, J. & Suttorp, M. 2009. Longitudinal Growth Retardation In A Prepubertal Girl With Chronic Myeloid Leukemia On Long-Term Treatment With Imatinib. *Hematologica,* 94, 1177-1179.

[49] Shah, N. P., Tran, C., Lee, F. Y., Chen, P., Norris, D. & Sawyers, C. L. 2004. Overriding Imatinib Resistance With A Novel Abl Kinase Inhibitor. *Science,* 305, 399-401.

[50] Shiang, R., Thompson, L. M., Zhu, Y. Z., Church, D. M., Fielder, T. J., Bocian, M., Winokur, S. T. & Wasmuth, J. J. 1994. Mutations In The Transmembrane Domain Of Fgfr3 Cause The Most Common Genetic Form Of Dwarfism, Achondroplasia. *Cell,* 78, 335-42.

[51] Shima, H., Tokuyama, M., Tanizawa, A., Tono, C., Hamamoto, K., Muramatsu, H., Watanabe, A., Hotta, N., Ito, M., Kurosawa, H., Kato, K., Tsurusawa, M., Horibe, K. & Shimada, H. 2011. Distinct Impact Of Imatinib On Growth At Prepubertal And Pubertal Ages Of Children With Chronic Myeloid Leukemia. *The Journal Of Pediatrics,* 159, 676-81.

[52] Suttorp, M. 2008. Innovative Approaches Of Targeted Therapy For Cml Of Childhood In Combination With Pediatric Hematopoietic Sct. *Bone Marrow Transplantation,* 42 Suppl 2, S40-6.

[53] Suttorp, M. & Millot, F. 2010. Treatment Of Pediatric Chronic Myeloid Leukemia In The Year 2010: Use Of Tyrosine Kinase Inhibitors And Stem-Cell Transplantation. *Hematology / The Education Program Of The American Society Of Hematology. American Society Of Hematology. Education Program,* 2010, 368-76.

[54] Suttorp, M., Thiede, C., Tauer, J. T., Roettgers, S., Sedlacek, P. & Harbott, J. 2009. Chronic Myeloid Leukemia In Pediatrics - First Results From Study Cml-Paed Ii [Abstract]. *Blood,* 114, 342.

[55] Tavormina, P. L., Rimoin, D. L., Cohn, D. H., Zhu, Y.-Z., Shiang, R. & Wasmuth, J. J. 1995. Another Mutation That Results In The Substitution Of An Unpaired Cysteine Residue In The Extracellular Domain Of Fgfr3 In Thanatophoric Dysplasia Type I. *Hum Mol Genet,* 4, 2175-7.

[56] Tibullo, D., Giallongo, C., La Cava, P., Berretta, S., Stagno, F., Chiarenza, A., Conticello, C., Palumbo, G. A. & Di Raimondo, F. 2009. Effects Of Imatinib Mesylate In Osteoblastogenesis. *Exp Hematol,* 37, 461-8.

[57] Tichelli, A., Rovo, A., Passweg, J., Schwarze, C. P., Van Lint, M. T., Arat, M. & Socie, G. 2009. Late Complications After Hematopoietic Stem Cell Transplantation. *Expert Review Of Hematology,* 2, 583-601.

[58] Vandyke, K., Dewar, A. L., Diamond, P., Fitter, S., Schultz, C. G., Sims, N. A. & Zannettino, A. C. W. 2010a. The Tyrosine Kinase Inhibitor Dasatinib Dysregulates Bone Remodeling Through Inhibition Of Osteoclasts *In Vivo*. *J Bone Miner Res,* 25, 1759-70.

[59] Vandyke, K., Dewar, A. L., Farrugia, A. N., Fitter, S., Bik To, L., Hughes, T. P. & Zannettino, A. C. W. 2009a. Therapeutic Concentrations Of Dasatinib Inhibit *In Vitro* Osteoclastogenesis. *Leukemia,* 23, 994-7.

[60] Vandyke, K., Dewar, A. L., Fitter, S., Menicanin, D., To, L. B., Hughes, T. P. & Zannettino, A. C. W. 2009b. Imatinib Mesylate Causes Growth Plate Closure *In Vivo*. *Leukemia,* 23, 2155-9.

[61] Vandyke, K., Fitter, S., Dewar, A. L., Hughes, T. P. & Zannettino, A. C. W. 2010b. Dysregulation Of Bone Remodeling By Imatinib Mesylate. *Blood,* 115, 766-74.

[62] Vandyke, K., Fitter, S., Drew, J., Fukumoto, S., Schultz, C. G., Sims, N. A., Hughes, T. P. & Zannettino, A. C. W. 2013. Prospective Histomorphometric And Dxa Evaluation Of Bone Remodelling In Imatinib-Treated Cml Patients: Evidence For Site-Specific Skeletal Effects. *Journal Of Clinical Endocrinology And Metabolism,* 98, 67-76.

[63] Vandyke, K., Fitter, S. & Zannettino, A. C. W. 2011. The Tyrosine Kinase Inhibitor Dasatinib (Sprycel) Inhibits Chondrocyte Activity And Proliferation *Blood Cancer Journal,* 1.

[64] Villemure, I. & Stokes, I. A. 2009. Growth Plate Mechanics And Mechanobiology. A Survey Of Present Understanding. *J Biomech,* 42, 1793-803.

[65] Wihlidal, P., Karlic, H., Pfeilstocker, M., Klaushofer, K. & Varga, F. 2008. Imatinib Mesylate (Im)-Induced Growth Inhibition Is Associated With Production Of Spliced Osteocalcin-Mrna In Cell Lines. *Leuk Res,* 32, 437-43.

[66] Wilsman, N. J., Farnum, C. E., Leiferman, E. M., Fry, M. & Barreto, C. 1996. Differential Growth By Growth Plates As A Function Of Multiple Parameters Of Chondrocytic Kinetics. *J Orthop Res,* 14, 927-36.

[67] Woods, K. A. & Savage, M. O. 1996. Laron Syndrome: Typical And Atypical Forms. *Baillieres Clin Endocrinol Metab,* 10, 371-87.

[68] Zwaan, C. M., Rizzari, C., Mechinaud, F., Lancaster, D. L., Kearns, P. R., Lehrnbecher, T., Van Der Elden, V. H. J., Beverloo, H. B., Den Boer, M. L., Pieters, R., Rosenberg, J., Herdlicka, R., Derreumaux, D., Agrawal, S. & Baruchel, A. 2010. Dasatinib In Children And Adolescents With Relapsed Or Refractory Leukemia: Results Of The Ca180018 Phase 1 Dose-Escalation Study Of The Innovative Therapies For Children With Cancer (Itcc) Consortium. *Blood,* 116, 2265.

[69] Zwaan, M. C., Rizzari, C., Van Der Velden, V. H. J., Beverloo, B., Den Boer, M. L., Baruchel, A., Mechinaud, F., Lancaster, D., Matloub, Y., Derreumaux, D., Pieters, R. & Kearns, P. 2008. Dasatinib In Children And Adolescents With Relapsed Or Refractory Leukemia: Interim Results Of The Ca180-018 Phase I Study From The Itcc Consortium. *Blood,* 112, 3241.

In: Imatinib
Editors: Mojtaba Akhtari and Ihab Elhemaidi
ISBN: 978-1-62808-297-5

Chapter 8

Pro-Apoptotic Effects of Imatinib on Pulmonary Artery Smooth Muscle Cells from Patients with Idiopathic Pulmonary Arterial Hypertension

Kazufumi Nakamura, Satoshi Akagi, Kusano Kengo, Aiko Ogawa, Hiromi Matsubara and Hiroshi Ito
Department of Cardiovascular Medicine,
Okayama University Graduate School of Medicine,
Dentistry and Pharmaceutical Sciences, Okayama, Japan

Abstract

Idiopathic pulmonary arterial hypertension (IPAH) is a progressive disease characterized by progressive elevation of pulmonary vascular resistance and pulmonary artery pressure. Remodeling of the pulmonary artery by an inappropriate increase of pulmonary artery smooth muscle cells (PASMCs) is problematic in the treatment of IPAH. Effective treatment that achieves reverse remodeling is required. This will require anti-proliferative and pro-apoptotic agents for PASMCs. We have reported that platelet-derived growth factor (PDGF)-BB stimulation causes a higher growth rate of cultured PASMCs from patients with IPAH than that of control cells. Therefore, we assessed anti-proliferative and pro-apoptotic effects of imatinib, a PDGF-receptor tyrosine kinase inhibitor, on cultured PASMCs obtained from IPAH. Treatment with imatinib (0.1 to 10 μg/mL) significantly inhibited PDGF-BB (10 ng/mL)-induced proliferation of PASMCs from IPAH patients. Imatinib (1 μg/mL) did not induce apoptosis in quiescent IPAH-PASMCs, but it had a pro-apoptotic effect on IPAH-PASMCs stimulated with PDGF-BB. Imatinib did not induce apoptosis in normal control PASMCs with or without PDGF-BB stimulation. PDGF-BB induced phosphorylation of Akt at 15 minutes, and Akt phosphorylation was inhibited by imatinib in IPAH-PASMCs. Akt-I-1/2 (1 μmol/L), an Akt inhibitor, in the presence of PDGF-BB significantly increased apoptotic cells compared with the control condition. Thus, Akt-I-1/2 could mimic the effects of imatinib on PASMCs.

In conclusion, imatinib has anti-proliferative and pro-apoptotic effects on IPAH-PASMCs stimulated with PDGF. The inhibitory effect of imatinib on Akt phosphorylation induced by PDGF plays an important role in the anti-proliferative and pro-apoptotic effects. Inhibition of PDGF signaling by imatinib may become a useful molecular-targeted therapy for IPAH.

Introduction

Idiopathic pulmonary arterial hypertension (IPAH) is a progressive disease characterized by progressive elevation of pulmonary vascular resistance (PVR) and pulmonary artery pressure. Increased PVR is induced by pulmonary vasoconstriction, vascular remodeling by intimal and medial hypertrophy, and thrombosis (Figure 1) [1, 2]. Pulmonary vascular medial hypertrophy is caused by an inappropriate increase in pulmonary artery smooth muscle cells (PASMCs). Treatment with several vasodilators such as calcium channel blockers, prostaglandin I_2 and endothelin receptor antagonists was found to improve survival of patients with IPAH, but 5-year survival remains at 50% [3, 4]. Effective treatment that achieves reverse remodeling is needed. This will require anti-proliferative and pro-apoptotic agents for PASMCs.

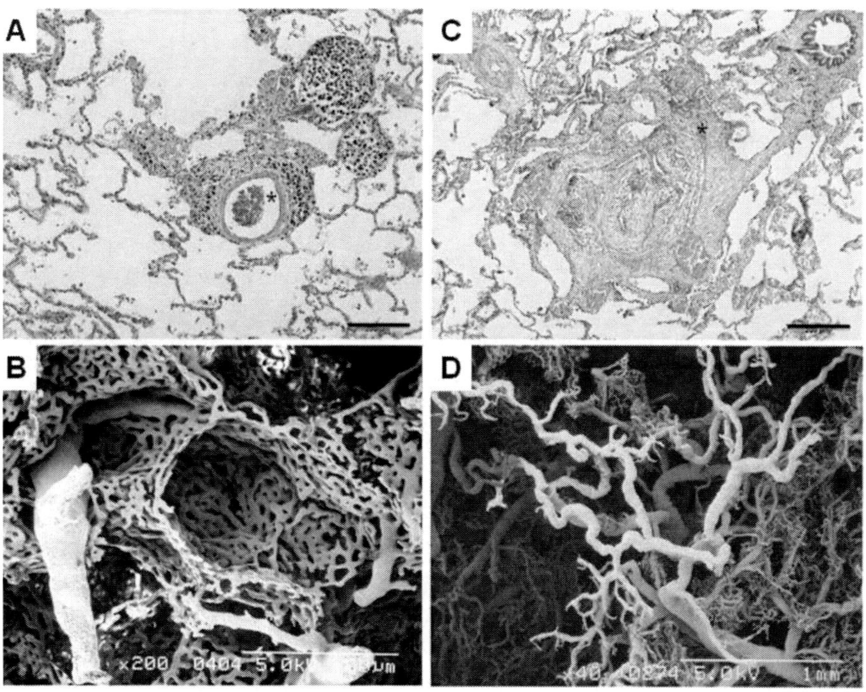

Figure 1. Images of microvessels from a normal control subject and a patients with idiopathic pulmonary arterial hypertension (Reference [2]). A. Hematoxylin-eosin staining of a small pulmonary artery (*). Bar = 200 μm. B. Scanning electron micrograph of blood vascular casts. Bar = 200 μm. C. Hematoxylin-eosin staining of small pulmonary arteries (*). Bar = 200 μm. D. Scanning electron micrograph of blood vascular casts. A deficient capillary network is seen. Bar = 1 mm.

We have reported that platelet-derived growth factor (PDGF)-BB stimulation causes a higher growth rate of cultured PASMCs from patients with IPAH than that of control cells (Figure 2A) [5-8]. PDGF-BB also increases the migration distance of IPAH-PASMCs compared with that of normal PASMCs significantly[7]. Recently, the use of a PDGF-receptor inhibitor such as imatinib (STI571) is starting to garner attention as a targeted therapy for pulmonary hypertension (PH) [9-12]. Imatinib is a drug used to treat certain types of cancer such as chronic myelogenous leukemia and gastrointestinal stromal tumors. In laboratory settings, imatinib is used as an experimental agent to suppress PDGF by inhibiting PDGF receptor ß (PDGF-Rß). It is an agent that acts by specifically inhibiting a certain enzyme, tyrosine kinase, that is characteristic of a particular cancer cell, rather than non-specifically inhibiting the proliferation of and killing all rapidly dividing cells. Schermuly et al reported that imatinib reverses pulmonary vascular remodeling and cor pulmonale in rats with monocrotaline-induced PH and in mice with chronic hypoxia-induced PH [9]. Perros et al reported that PDGF-BB-induced proliferation and migration of PASMCs from patients with IPAH were inhibited by imatinib [11].

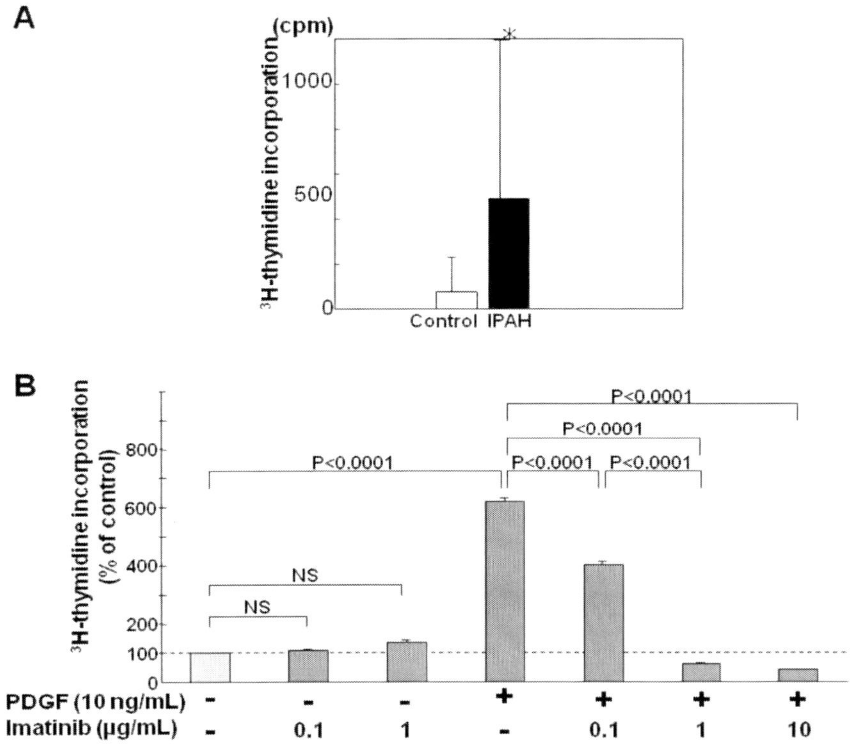

Figure 2. Effects of PDGF and imatinib on proliferation of pulmonary artery smooth muscle cells (PASMCs) (Reference [5] and [13]). A. Comparison of PDGF-stimulated proliferation of on PASMCs of the control patients and patients with idiopathic pulmonary arterial hypertension (IPAH) (Reference [5]). ^{3}H-thymidine incorporation was measured as counts per minute (cpm). Data are mean ± SE of patients with IPAH and 5 control patients. *P<0.05 compared with control. B. Inhibitory effect of imatinib on proliferation of PASMCs from IPAH patients (Reference [13]). Anti-proliferative effects of imatinib (0.1 to 10 µg/mL) on IPAH-PASMCs stimulated with PDGF-BB (10 ng/mL). ^{3}H-thymidine incorporation was measured. Counts per minute (cpm) were expressed as a percentage of cpm of IPAH-PASMCs treated with a diluent (control). Data are mean ± SE.

Not only inhibition of proliferation but also induction of apoptosis of PASMCs is needed to actively reduce stenosis due to vascular remodeling at small pulmonary arteries of patients with IPAH. These two effects may lead to reverse remodeling of the pulmonary vasculature. Expression of PDGF-B is up-regulated in the medial layer of small pulmonary arteries of rats with monocrotaline-induced PH and imatinib induces apoptosis in the small pulmonary arteries [9]. However, imatinib does not induce apoptosis in cultured IPAH-PASMCs without PDGF treatment [11]. Thus, imatinib may not be able to induce apoptosis in quiescent cells. We hypothesized that imatinib in the presence of PDGF-BB induces apoptosis of PASMCs from patients with IPAH, but that imatinib can not induce apoptosis in PASMCs without PDGF stimulation. We therefore investigated whether imatinib in the presence and absence of PDGF-BB induces apoptosis of PASMCs from patients with IPAH [13].

Akt is a member of the serine/threonine-specific kinase family known for facilitating cell survival via inhibition of apoptotic pathways [14]. Therefore, induction of apoptosis of IPAH-PASMCs may be related to Akt inactivation. We also investigated whether imatinib inhibits Akt activation [13].

Materials and Methods

Isolation, Culture and Identification of Pasmcs

Peripheral segments of the pulmonary artery were obtained at lung transplantation [15] from 8 patients with IPAH as previously described [13, 16] (2 males and 6 females; mean age, 22±4 years; age range 11-43 years) . For normal control experiments, samples of pulmonary arteries were also obtained at lung lobectomy from a patient with bronchogenic carcinoma (male, 58 years old) who showed no evidence of PAH and received no systemic chemotherapy or radiation therapy before lung lobectomy as previously described [5, 6, 8, 13, 16]. Samples of the pulmonary arteries were obtained from the most distal area from the carcinoma in the resected lobe.

All of the studies were approved by the Ethics Committee of Okayama University Graduate School of Medicine, Density, and Pharmaceutical Sciences, and written informed consent was obtained from all patients before the procedure. The investigation also conforms to the principles outlined in the Declaration of Helsinki.

PASMCs were isolated as described previously [5, 6, 8, 16, 17]. Peripheral segments of pulmonary arteries smaller than 1 mm in outer diameter were disaggregated with collagenase and cut into 2-mm-long sections, and then the adventitia and endothelial cell layers were removed. Vessels were plated on a 6-well plate with Dulbecco's modified Eagle's medium (DMEM) supplemented with 10% fetal bovine serum (FBS) and 0.1 mg/mL kanamycin and incubated in a humidified 5% CO2 atmosphere at 37°C. The culture medium was changed every 3 days. After reaching confluence, the cells were subcultured by treatment with trypsin 0.05%)/ethylenediaminetetraacetic acid (EDTA) (0.02%). Cell identification was confirmed by examination of cytoskeletal components (α-smooth muscle actin and myosin) using an immunocytochemical technique as described previously [16]. Cells between passages 3 to 5 were used for all experiments.

Evaluation of Apoptosis

TUNEL assays were performed using an ApopTag fluorescein in situ apoptosis detection kit (Chemicon International Inc.) according to the manufacturer's instructions as described previously [13, 18]. Nuclear morphology was examined by labeling with DAPI solution (0.6 μg/mL, Dojindo Laboratories). Immunofluorescence staining was performed to confirm α-smooth muscle actin (αSMA) expression using αSMA antibody (1:100 dilution, Sigma). Caspase assay was performed using a CaspaTag Caspase-3/7 in situ apoptosis detection kit (Chemicon International Inc.) according to the manufacturer's instructions. Nuclear morphology was examined by Hoechst staining. The samples were analyzed by fluorescence microscopy (Olympus IX71, Olympus Optical Co. Ltd, Tokyo, Japan). For each cover slip, 5-10 fields (with 10-30 cells in each field) were randomly selected to determine the percentage of apoptotic cells in total cells based on the morphological characteristics of apoptosis. PASMCs were reseeded on collagen-coated glass cover slips in 12-well plates at a density of 5×10^4 cells/well on day 0. After 16 hours of incubation (on day 1), the culture media were replaced with low-serum culture media (DMEM, 0.1% FBS, and 0.1 mg/mL kanamycin), and the cultured cells were made quiescent for 48 hours. On day 3, PDGF-BB (10 ng/mL), imatinib (1 μg/mL) or Akt-I-1/2 (1 μmol/L) was added to the media. After 24 hours (on day 4), the cells were stained by using an ApopTag fluorescein in situ apoptosis detection kit or CaspaTag in situ apoptosis detection kit.

Results

Inhibitory Effect of Imatinib on Proliferation of Pasmcs from IPAH Patients

Treatment with imatinib inhibited PDGF-BB-induced proliferation of PASMCs from IPAH patients as assessed by ^{3}H-thymidine incorporation (n = 5-12 experiments in each cell) (Figure 2B). This result is consistent with recent findings of other investigators [11].

Effect of Imatinib on Apoptosis of Pasmcs from IPAH Patients

We performed a TUNEL assay using an ApopTag fluorescein to assess the effect of imatinib on apoptosis of PASMCs from IPAH patients as described previously [13]. Figure 3A shows representative cases of the TUNEL assay. TUNEL-positive cell (green) was observed after 24-hour treatment with imatinib (1 μg/mL) in the presence of PDGF-BB (10 ng/mL) (Figure 3D and H). However, imatinib (1 μg/mL) (Figure 3B and F) or PDGF-BB (10 ng/mL) (Figure 3C and G) alone did not induce apoptosis in IPAH-PASMCs. Imatinib (1 μg/mL) in the presence of PDGF-BB (10 ng/mL) significantly increased TUNEL-positive cells in IPAH-PASMCs compared with the control condition in IPAH-PASMCs ($P < 0.05$: 15.1±5.4% versus 4.5±1.3%, n = 4 or 5 experiments in each cell line) (Figure 3J). There was no significant difference in the percentage of TUNEL-positive cells between the imatinib alone or PDGF alone condition and the control condition (Figure 3J). There was also no significant difference between the imatinib alone, PDGF alone or both imatinib and PDGF condition and the control condition in normal PASMCs (P = NS, n = 5 experiments) (Figure 3I).

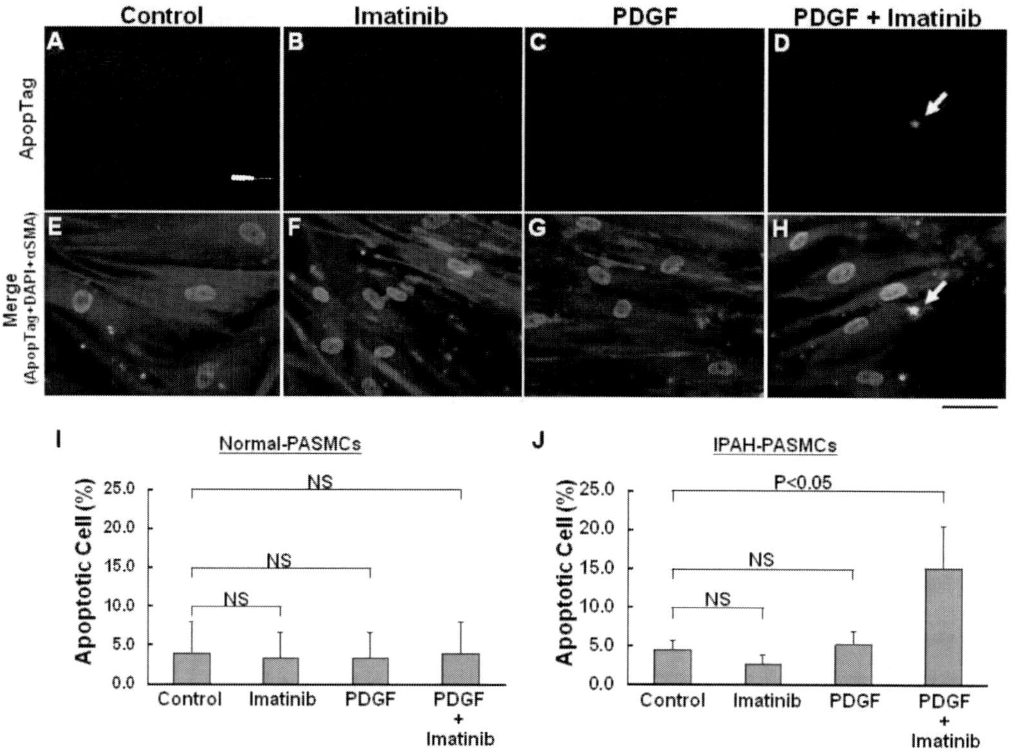

Figure 3. Effect of imatinib on apoptosis of pulmonary artery smooth muscle cells (PASMCs) of idiopathic pulmonary arterial hypertension (IPAH) in TUNEL assay by ApopTag fluorescein (Reference [13]). A to D, ApopTag fluorescein (green). E to H, Combined images (merge) of ApopTag fluorescein, DAPI nuclear staining (blue) and alpha smooth muscle actin (αSMA) (red). A and E, IPAH-PASMCs without treatment. B and F, IPAH-PASMCs treated with imatinib (1 μg/mL). C and G, IPAH-PASMCs treated with PDGF-BB (10 ng/mL). D and H, IPAH-PASMCs treated with imatinib and PDGF-BB. Arrow shows a TUNEL-positive cell (green). Bar = 500 μm. I, Effect of imatinib on apoptosis of normal PASMCs in TUNEL assay. J, Effect of imatinib on apoptosis of IPAH-PASMCs in TUNEL assay. Imatinib (1 μg/mL) in the presence of PDGF-BB (10 ng/mL) significantly increased TUNEL-positive (apoptotic) cells in IPAH-PASMCs compared with the control condition (P<0.05). Data are mean ± SE.

Figure 4 shows representative cases of the caspase assay in IPAH-PASMCs. Caspase-3 and -7-active cell was observed after 24-hour treatment with imatinib (1 μg/mL) in the presence of PDGF-BB (10 ng/mL) (Figure 4D and H). Imatinib (1 μg/mL) in the presence of PDGF-BB (10 ng/mL) significantly increased caspase-3 and -7-active cells in IPAH-PASMCs compared with the control condition (P <0.01: 12.4±3.0% versus 2.2±1.2 %, n = 5 experiments in each cell line) (Figure 4J). There was no significant difference in the percentage of caspase-3 and -7-positive cells between the imatinib alone or PDGF alone condition and the control condition in IPAH-PASMCs (Figure 4J). There was also no significant difference between the imatinib alone, PDGF alone or both imatinib and PDGF condition and the control condition in normal PASMCs (P = NS, n = 5 experiments) (Figure 4I).

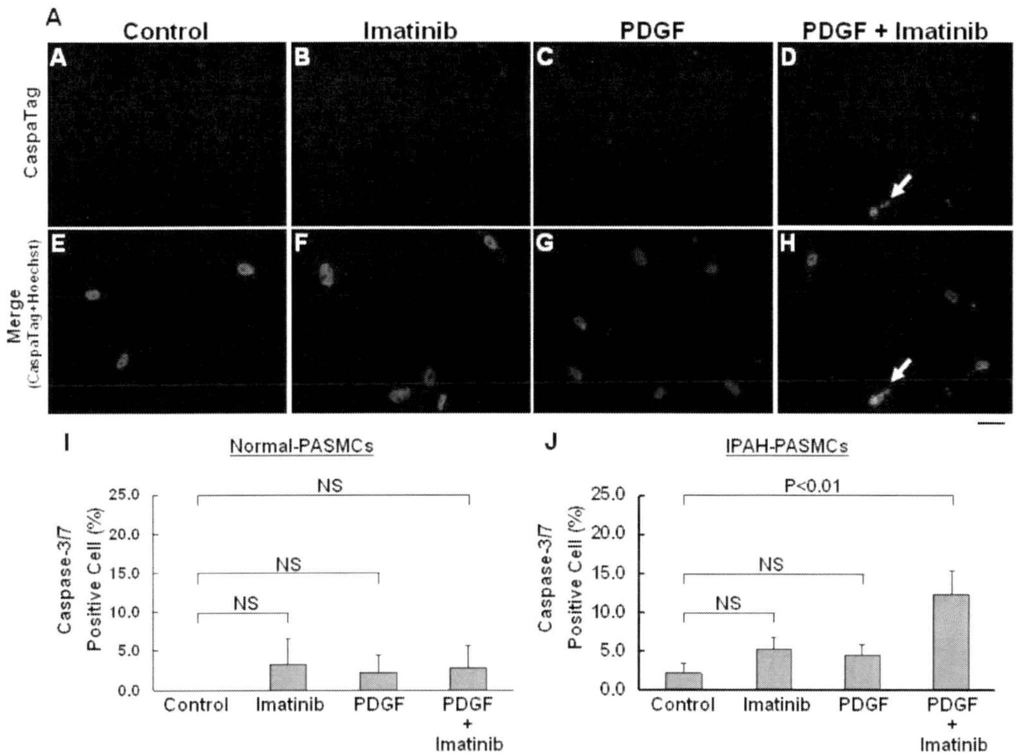

Figure 4. Effect of imatinib on apoptosis of pulmonary artery smooth muscle cells (PASMCs) of idiopathic pulmonary arterial hypertension (IPAH) in Caspase assay using a CaspaTag Caspase-3/7 in situ apoptosis detection kit (Reference [13]). A to D, CaspaTag staining (green). E to H, Combined images (merge) of CaspaTag staining and Hoechst nuclear staining (blue). A and E, IPAH-PASMCs without treatment. B and F, IPAH-PASMCs treated with imatinib (1 μg/mL). C and G, IPAH-PASMCs treated with PDGF-BB (10 ng/mL). D and H, IPAH-PASMCs treated with imatinib and PDGF-BB. Arrow shows a caspase-3/7-positive cell (green). Bar = 500 μm. I, Effect of imatinib on apoptosis of normal PASMCs in Caspase assay. J, Effect of imatinib on apoptosis of IPAH-PASMCs in Caspase assay. Imatinib (1 μg/mL) in the presence of PDGF-BB (10 ng/mL) significantly increased caspase-positive (apoptotic) cells in IPAH-PASMCs compared with the control condition ($P<0.01$). Data are mean ± SE.

These results show that imatinib did not induce apoptosis in normal PASMCs and quiescent IPAH-PASMCs but that imatinib had a proapoptotic effect on IPAH-PASMCs stimulated with PDGF.

Effect of Imatinib on PDGF-BB-Induced Phosphorylation of Akt

Western blot analysis revealed that PDGF-BB induced phosphorylation of Akt at 15 minutes (Figure 5A, lanes 2 and B). Akt phosphorylation was significantly inhibited by imatinib (1 ng/mL) compared with treatment with PDGF-BB ($P < 0.05$, n = 4 experiments) (Figure 5A, lanes 3 and B).

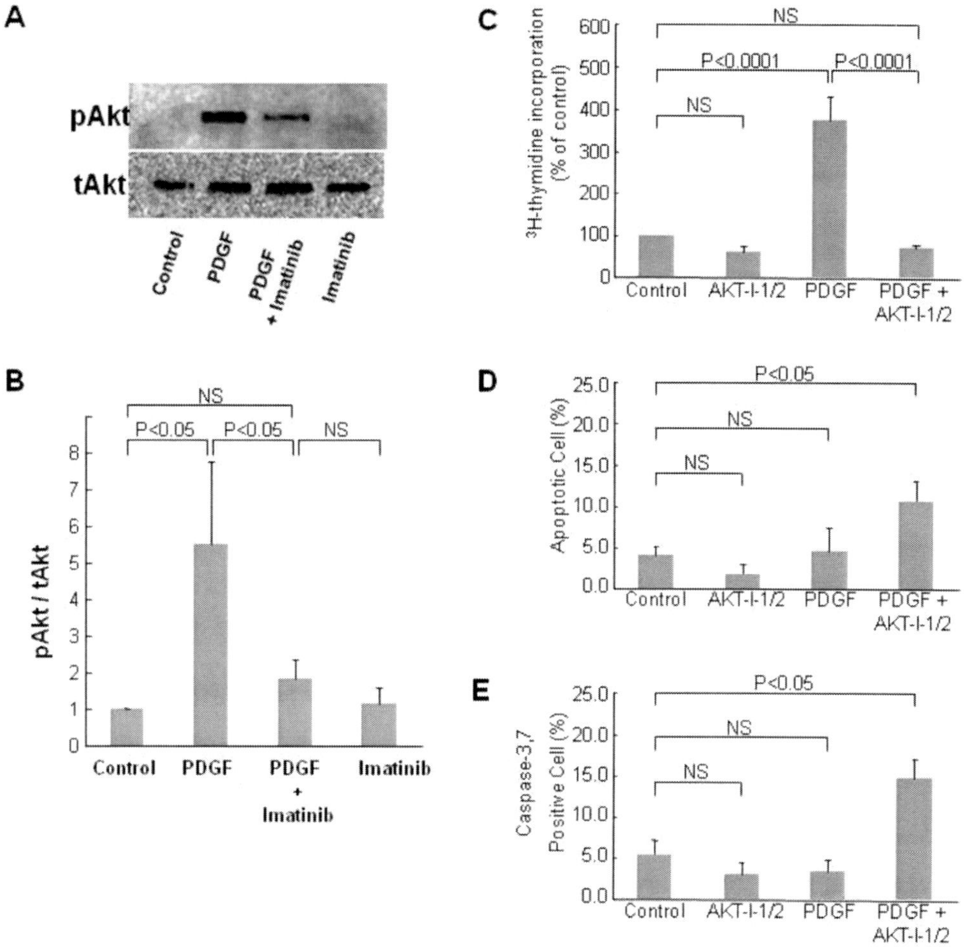

Figure 5. Effect of imatinib on PDGF-BB-induced phosphorylation of Akt and effects of an Akt inhibitor on PDGF-BB-stimulated proliferation and apoptosis of pulmonary artery smooth muscle cells (PASMCs) of idiopathic pulmonary arterial hypertension (IPAH) (Reference [13]). A, Western blot analysis of total Akt (tAkt) and phosphorylated Akt (pAkt). PDGF-BB (10 ng/mL) induced phosphorylation of Akt at 15 minutes (lanes 2). Akt phosphorylation was inhibited by imatinib (1 ng/mL) (lanes 3). B, Bar graphs show semiquantitive analysis of pAkt expression level in IPAH-PASMCs. Data are mean ± SE of the intensity of the band corresponding to pAkt relative to tAkt. C, Anti-proliferative effect of Akt-I-1/2 (1 μmol/L), an Akt inhibitor, on IPAH-PASMCs stimulated with PDGF-BB (10 ng/mL). ^{3}H-thymidine incorporation was measured. Counts per minute (cpm) were expressed as a percentage of cpm of IPAH-PASMCs treated with a diluent (control). Data are mean ± SE. D, Effect of Akt-I-1/2 (1 μmol/L) on apoptosis of PASMCs in TUNEL assay by ApopTag fluorescein. E, Effect of Akt-I-1/2 (1 μmol/L) on apoptosis of PASMCs in Caspase assay using a CaspaTag Caspase-3/7 in situ apoptosis detection kit.

Akt-I-1/2 (1 μmol/L), an Akt inhibitor, could mimic the effects of imatinib on PASMCs. Akt-I-1/2 significantly inhibited PDGF-induced proliferation of IPAH-PASMCs as assessed by ^{3}H-thymidine incorporation ($P < 0.001$, n = 10 experiments) (Figure 5C). Akt-I-1/2 in the presence of PDGF-BB significantly increased TUNEL-positive cells ($P < 0.05$, n = 5 experiments) (Figure 5D) and caspase-3,7-positive cells in IPAH-PASMCs ($P < 0.05$, n = 5 experiments) (Figure 5E) compared with the control condition. These results show that inhibition of Akt is strongly related to anti-proliferative and pro-apoptotic effects of imatinib on PDGF-stimulated IPAH-PASMCs.

Discussion

Two major new findings were obtained in the present study as previously described [13]. First, imatinib did not induce apoptosis in quiescent IPAH-PASMCs and normal PASMCs, but it had a pro-apoptotic effect on IPAH-PASMCs stimulated with PDGF. Second, inhibition of Akt is related to the anti-proliferative and pro-apoptotic effects of imatinib on PDGF-stimulated IPAH-PASMCs.

Imatinib alone did not induce apoptosis in IPAH-PASMCs. This result is consistent with recent findings of other investigators [11]. However, the combination of imatinib and PDGF induced apoptosis. Therefore, imatinib did not induce apoptosis in quiescent IPAH-PASMCs, but it had a pro-apoptotic effect on IPAH-PASMCs stimulated with PDGF. It has been reported that PDGF-A and PDGF-B mRNA levels were increased in small pulmonary arteries from patients with IPAH [11] and that serum PDGF-BB levels across the lung circulation were higher in IPAH patients [19]. Therefore, imatinib is expected to induce apoptosis in clinical settings. Further studies are needed to clarify this point.

Recent clinical trial suggested the safety and the efficacy of imatinib in patients with PAH 20-22. A double-blind, placebo-controlled, multicenter phase II trial of imatinib in patients with PAH (NCT00477269) suggested that hemodynamic measurement were in favor of imatinib 20. According to a recent press release 22, a double-blind, placebo-controlled multicenter phase III trial (IMPRES; NCT00902174) showed significantly improved walking distance in patients with life-threatening pulmonary arterial hypertension. These beneficial effects might be influenced by reverse-remodeling effect of imatinib in pulmonary artery. It is hoped more evidence of reverse-remodeling effect of imatinib will be revealed.

Many signaling pathways, including ERK, p38 MAPK and Akt, are involved in proliferation and survival of PASMCs [8, 23]. Akt is a member of the serine/threonine-specific kinase family known for facilitating cell survival via inhibition of apoptotic pathways. It has been shown that PDGF stimulation transiently phosphorylates Akt and the mammalian target of rapamycin (mTOR) in PASMCs from patients with chronic thromboembolic pulmonary hypertension [23]. In our study, PDGF-BB induced phosphorylation of Akt and it was inhibited by imatinib in IPAH-PASMCs. Akt-I-1/2, an Akt inhibitor, could mimic the effects of imatinib on PASMCs. Akt is related to the anti-proliferative and pro-apoptotic effects of imatinib on PDGF-stimulated IPAH-PASMCs.

Imatinib is a drug used for treating chronic myelogenous leukemia and gastrointestinal stromal tumors. However, resistance to imatinib can occur [24-26]. Not only primary resistance within the first two months but also secondary resistance develops after a median of about 2 years of treatment with the drug. Hatano et al reported that imatinib decreases the plasma concentration of PDGF-BB in patients with PAH [12]. We showed that imatinib had a pro-apoptotic effect on IPAH-PASMCs stimulated with PDGF in the present study. Thus, imatinib would induce apoptosis only in the early period of treatment when plasma PDGF-BB levels are relatively high. After the PDGF levels have decreased, imatinib would not be able to induce apoptosis. Therefore, resistance to imatinib might occur in patients with pulmonary hypertension. Attention may be needed in clinical use.

Conclusion

Imatinib inhibited PDGF-induced proliferation of IPAH-PASMCs. Imatinib did not induce apoptosis in quiescent IPAH-PASMCs, but it had a pro-apoptotic effect on IPAH-PASMCs stimulated with PDGF. Inhibition of Akt may be important in the anti-proliferative and pro-apoptotic effects of imatinib on PDGF-stimulated IPAH-PASMCs. Modulation of PDGF signaling such as Akt is important. Inhibition of PDGF signaling by imatinib may become a useful molecular-targeted therapy for IPAH.

References

[1] Archer S, Rich S. Primary pulmonary hypertension: A vascular biology and translational research "work in progress". *Circulation*. 2000;102(22):2781-2791

[2] Miura A, Nakamura K, Kusano KF, Matsubara H, Ogawa A, Akagi S, Oto T, Murakami T, Ohtsuka A, Yutani C, Ohe T, Ito H. Three-dimensional structure of pulmonary capillary vessels in patients with pulmonary hypertension. *Circulation*. 2010;121(19):2151-2153

[3] Barst RJ. Pdgf signaling in pulmonary arterial hypertension. *J Clin Invest*. 2005;115(10):2691-2694

[4] Barst RJ, Gibbs JS, Ghofrani HA, Hoeper MM, McLaughlin VV, Rubin LJ, Sitbon O, Tapson VF, Galie N. Updated evidence-based treatment algorithm in pulmonary arterial hypertension. *J Am Coll Cardiol*. 2009;54(1 Suppl):S78-84

[5] Ogawa A, Nakamura K, Matsubara H, Fujio H, Ikeda T, Kobayashi K, Miyazaki I, Asanuma M, Miyaji K, Miura D, Kusano KF, Date H, Ohe T. Prednisolone inhibits proliferation of cultured pulmonary artery smooth muscle cells of patients with idiopathic pulmonary arterial hypertension. *Circulation*. 2005;112(12):1806-1812

[6] Fujio H, Nakamura K, Matsubara H, Kusano KF, Miyaji K, Nagase S, Ikeda T, Ogawa A, Ohta-Ogo K, Miura D, Miura A, Miyazaki M, Date H, Ohe T. Carvedilol inhibits proliferation of cultured pulmonary artery smooth muscle cells of patients with idiopathic pulmonary arterial hypertension. *J Cardiovasc Pharmacol*. 2006;47(2):250-255

[7] Ikeda T, Nakamura K, Akagi S, Kusano KF, Matsubara H, Fujio H, Ogawa A, Miura A, Miura D, Oto T, Yamanaka R, Otsuka F, Date H, Ohe T, Ito H. Inhibitory effects of simvastatin on platelet-derived growth factor signaling in pulmonary artery smooth muscle cells from patients with idiopathic pulmonary arterial hypertension. *J Cardiovasc Pharmacol*. 2010;55(1):39-48

[8] Takeda M, Otsuka F, Nakamura K, Inagaki K, Suzuki J, Miura D, Fujio H, Matsubara H, Date H, Ohe T, Makino H. Characterization of the bone morphogenetic protein (bmp) system in human pulmonary arterial smooth muscle cells isolated from a sporadic case of primary pulmonary hypertension: Roles of bmp type ib receptor

(activin receptor-like kinase-6) in the mitotic action. *Endocrinology*. 2004;145(9):4344-4354

[9] Schermuly RT, Dony E, Ghofrani HA, Pullamsetti S, Savai R, Roth M, Sydykov A, Lai YJ, Weissmann N, Seeger W, Grimminger F. Reversal of experimental pulmonary hypertension by pdgf inhibition. *J Clin Invest*. 2005;115(10):2811-2821

[10] Ghofrani HA, Seeger W, Grimminger F. Imatinib for the treatment of pulmonary arterial hypertension. *N Engl J Med*. 2005;353(13):1412-1413

[11] Perros F, Montani D, Dorfmuller P, Durand-Gasselin I, Tcherakian C, Le Pavec J, Mazmanian M, Fadel E, Mussot S, Mercier O, Herve P, Emilie D, Eddahibi S, Simonneau G, Souza R, Humbert M. Platelet-derived growth factor expression and function in idiopathic pulmonary arterial hypertension. *Am J Respir Crit Care Med*. 2008;178(1):81-88

[12] Hatano M, Yao A, Shiga T, Kinugawa K, Hirata Y, Nagai R. Imatinib mesylate has the potential to exert its efficacy by down-regulating the plasma concentration of platelet-derived growth factor in patients with pulmonary arterial hypertension. *Int Heart J*. 2010;51(4):272-276

[13] Nakamura K, Akagi S, Ogawa A, Kusano KF, Matsubara H, Miura D, Fuke S, Nishii N, Nagase S, Kohno K, Morita H, Oto T, Yamanaka R, Otsuka F, Miura A, Yutani C, Ohe T, Ito H. Pro-apoptotic effects of imatinib on pdgf-stimulated pulmonary artery smooth muscle cells from patients with idiopathic pulmonary arterial hypertension. *Int J Cardiol*. 2012;159(2):100-106

[14] Wendel HG, De Stanchina E, Fridman JS, Malina A, Ray S, Kogan S, Cordon-Cardo C, Pelletier J, Lowe SW. Survival signalling by akt and eif4e in oncogenesis and cancer therapy. *Nature*. 2004;428(6980):332-337

[15] Date H, Kusano KF, Matsubara H, Ogawa A, Fujio H, Miyaji K, Okazaki M, Yamane M, Toyooka S, Aoe M, Sano Y, Hanazaki M, Goto K, Kasahara S, Sano S, Ohe T. Living-donor lobar lung transplantation for pulmonary arterial hypertension after failure of epoprostenol therapy. *J Am Coll Cardiol*. 2007;50(6):523-527

[16] Nakamura K, Shimizu J, Kataoka N, Hashimoto K, Ikeda T, Fujio H, Ohta-Ogo K, Ogawa A, Miura A, Mohri S, Nagase S, Morita H, Kusano KF, Date H, Matsubara H, Mochizuki S, Hashimoto K, Kajiya F, Ohe T. Altered nano/micro-order elasticity of pulmonary artery smooth muscle cells of patients with idiopathic pulmonary arterial hypertension. *Int J Cardiol*. 2010;140(1):102-107

[17] Kouchi H, Nakamura K, Fushimi K, Sakaguchi M, Miyazaki M, Ohe T, Namba M. Manumycin a, inhibitor of ras farnesyltransferase, inhibits proliferation and migration of rat vascular smooth muscle cells. *Biochem Biophys Res Commun*. 1999;264(3):915-920

[18] Nikaido A, Tada T, Nakamura K, Murakami M, Banba K, Nishii N, Fuke S, Nagase S, Sakuragi S, Morita H, Ohe T, Kusano KF. Clinical features of and effects of angiotensin system antagonists on amiodarone-induced pulmonary toxicity. *Int J Cardiol*. 2010;140(3):328-335

[19] Selimovic N, Bergh CH, Andersson B, Sakiniene E, Carlsten H, Rundqvist B. Growth factors and interleukin-6 across the lung circulation in pulmonary hypertension. *Eur Respir J*. 2009;34(3):662-668

[20] Ghofrani HA, Morrell NW, Hoeper MM, Olschewski H, Peacock AJ, Barst RJ, Shapiro S, Golpon H, Toshner M, Grimminger F, Pascoe S. Imatinib in pulmonary arterial

hypertension patients with inadequate response to established therapy. *Am J Respir Crit Care Med.* 2010;182(9):1171-1177

[21] ten Freyhaus H, Dumitrescu D, Berghausen E, Vantler M, Caglayan E, Rosenkranz S. Imatinib mesylate for the treatment of pulmonary arterial hypertension. *Expert Opin Investig Drugs.* 2012;21(1):119-134

[22] Press release, Novartis Pharma. IMPRES trial. Data on file. 2011

[23] Ogawa A, Firth AL, Yao W, Madani MM, Kerr KM, Auger WR, Jamieson SW, Thistlethwaite PA, Yuan JX. Inhibition of mtor attenuates store-operated ca2+ entry in cells from endarterectomized tissues of patients with chronic thromboembolic pulmonary hypertension. *Am J Physiol Lung Cell Mol Physiol.* 2009;297(4):L666-676

[24] Kantarjian H, Giles F, Wunderle L, Bhalla K, O'Brien S, Wassmann B, Tanaka C, Manley P, Rae P, Mietlowski W, Bochinski K, Hochhaus A, Griffin JD, Hoelzer D, Albitar M, Dugan M, Cortes J, Alland L, Ottmann OG. Nilotinib in imatinib-resistant cml and philadelphia chromosome-positive all. *N Engl J Med.* 2006;354(24):2542-2551

[25] Demetri GD, von Mehren M, Blanke CD, Van den Abbeele AD, Eisenberg B, Roberts PJ, Heinrich MC, Tuveson DA, Singer S, Janicek M, Fletcher JA, Silverman SG, Silberman SL, Capdeville R, Kiese B, Peng B, Dimitrijevic S, Druker BJ, Corless C, Fletcher CD, Joensuu H. Efficacy and safety of imatinib mesylate in advanced gastrointestinal stromal tumors. *N Engl J Med.* 2002;347(7):472-480

[26] Verweij J, Casali PG, Zalcberg J, LeCesne A, Reichardt P, Blay JY, Issels R, van Oosterom A, Hogendoorn PC, Van Glabbeke M, Bertulli R, Judson I. Progression-free survival in gastrointestinal stromal tumours with high-dose imatinib: Randomised trial. *Lancet.* 2004;364(9440):1127-1134

In: Imatinib
Editors: Mojtaba Akhtari and Ihab Elhemaidi

ISBN: 978-1-62808-297-5

Chapter 9

Secondary Molecular Targets of Imatinib in Cancer Cells

Germana Rappa and Aurelio Lorico
Cancer Research Program, Roseman University of Health Sciences,
Las Vegas, NV, US

Abstract

Imatinib mesylate (Imatinib) has been the first approved drug, under the commercial name of Gleevec, to directly turn off the signal of a protein known to cause cancer. The story of Imatinib is a beautiful example of how knowledge of the biological functioning of a cell can lead to life-saving medical treatment. It was rationally designed in the laboratory to target a peculiar tyrosine kinase, the oncogenic Bcr-Abl gene fusion product, consequent to the t(9;22)(q34;q11) chromosomal translocation, extremely common in chronic myeloid leukemia (CML). Although it does not eradicate CML cells, it does greatly limit the growth of the tumor clone and decreases the risk of blast crisis. The efficacy of Imatinib in CML may be explained by the fact that while most cancers are caused by a multitude of complex interacting genetic and environmental factors, CML is mainly caused by a single aberrant protein, Bcr-Abl. Nonetheless, there has been increasing interest in understanding other potential targets of Imatinib to evaluate the specificity, safety and potential off-target effects of this first-in-class drug. Several studies have demonstrated that Imatinib is not entirely selective: it also inhibits the receptor tyrosine kinases for platelet-derived growth factor (PDGF), stem cell factor (SCF), and c-KIT, as well as PDGF and SCF-mediated cellular events. It has been proposed that dual BCR-ABL/c-KIT inhibition may be important to suppress the majority of CML cell types that rely on both BCR-ABL and c-KIT activity. The lack of specificity of Imatinib has been exploited in the clinic, leading to approved use for the treatment of chronic eosinophilic leukemia, caused by a FIP1L1-PDGFR-alpha fusion kinase, and for gastrointestinal stromal tumors, caused by mutations of *c-KIT* or *PDGFR-alpha*. Vacuolar H(+)-ATPase, an evolutionarily conserved proton pump, and NAD(P)H dehydrogenase, quinone 2, have also been identified as additional targets. In human MA-11 breast carcinoma cells, expressing both ABL and PDGFR, Imatinib selected cells with increased motility and aggressive behavior. Also, intraperitoneal treatment of MA-11 xenografts with Imatinib did not result in an antitumor effect, but rather increased the tumor take rate and caused the appearance of large abdominal masses in 30% of mice. Identification of all the molecular players that are involved in Imatinib activity, and assessment of their relative importance *in vivo* will lead to a refinement of its clinical spectrum of efficacy.

Introduction

Chronic myeloid leukemia (CML), a malignancy where the Abelson (ABL) gene is constitutively activated by fusion with the BCR gene (BCR-ABL), is the archetypical disease, in which imatinib mesylate (Imatinib) has acquired therapeutic relevance [1, 2]. Imatinib is a selective small protein kinase inhibitor that targets the ABL tyrosine kinase, and inhibits the growth of BCR-ABL expressing chronic myeloid leukemia (CML) progenitor cells, by blockade of the adenosine triphosphate (ATP)-binding site of the tyrosine kinase domain of the oncogenic BCR-ABL fusion protein. Despite toxicity problems and occurrence of drug resistance, the success of Imatinib in the treatment of CML remains the best example of successful targeted therapy. However, as presented in this review, Imatinib is not entirely specific and targets tyrosine kinases other than ABL, as well as proteins devoid of kinase activity. While off-target effects may result in undesirable collateral toxicity, they also lead to potential synergism and additional clinical indications for Imatinib.

c-KIT and PDGFR-Alpha

A gain-of-function mutation of *c-KIT* or *PDGFR-alpha* is the crucial step in tumorigenesis of gastro-intestinal stromal tumors (GIST), the most common mesenchymal tumors of the gastrointestinal tract. Imatinib can block the activated receptor kinase activity of both c-KIT and PDGFR-alpha. Advanced cases of GIST, in which margin-negative-resection can not be reached, can be successfully treated with Imatinib at doses of 400 mg/day, with objective responses reached in more than 50% of patients [3]. Furthermore, even in those patients with stable disease, long-term tumor control can be achieved. Imatinib is also indicated for treatment of metastatic GIST and, since 2012, for adjuvant treatment of adult patients following complete gross resection of c-KIT$^+$ GIST. Based on the result of a retrospective analysis, Imatinib as a single agent is also a treatment option for patients with recurrent meningiomas with prevalent expression of PDGF receptors [4].

Recent studies have provided mechanistic insight into how c-KIT/PDGFR-alpha kinase inhibition leads to clinical responses in GIST patients, and have established the soluble histone H2AX as a novel target in cancer therapy. Histones form the so-called nucleosome, around which DNA is wrapped. More recently, a plethora of novel functions of histones have been discovered, including a role of histone H2AX in the signaling cascades that are activated after the cellular DNA is damaged. In fact, non-nucleosomal H2AX is induced by DNA replication stress and sensitizes cells to undergo apoptosis by aberrant chromatin aggregation, leading to transcriptional block [5]. Imatinib induces C-terminal phosphorylation of H2AX at Ser139 and Tyr142 and subsequent apoptosis in BCR-ABL-positive K562 cells via the caspase-3/MST1 pathway [6]. Interestingly, Imatinib-mediated H2AX up-regulation correlated with Imatinib sensitivity, while depletion of H2AX attenuated the apoptotic response of GIST cells to Imatinib [7].

In neurofibromatosis, the finding of the importance of mast cell recruitment via c-KIT signaling suggested the possible clinical utility of Imatinib in this syndrome, by inhibiting mast cell recruitment and the subsequent matrix formation and angiogenesis required for the development of neurofibromas [8]. These findings have resulted in two pilot clinical studies to determine the efficacy of Imatinib in neurofibromatosis patients with plexiform neurofibromas.

Primary and metastatic uveal melanoma is a condition in which prevalent expression of c-KIT and of its ligand SCF are found. So, c-KIT may be a potential target for therapy with Imatinib in these melanomas. Studies by Hofmann [9] have been disappointing in this regard, showing that over-expression of c-KIT/SCF in uveal melanoma does not translate into clinical efficacy of Imatinib, suggesting a more complicated spectrum of mechanism of action of Imatinib on c-KIT. The observation that, by blocking the abnormal activation of PDGFR signaling, Imatinib reduced the disruption of the elastic layer, smooth muscle cell proliferation, and aneurysm formation supports a potential clinical utility of Imatinib in the prevention of atherosclerosis [10].

FIP1L1-PDGFR-Alpha

The lack of Imatinib specificity has been further exploited in the clinics, with Imatinib gaining approval for the treatment of chronic eosinophilic leukemia (CEL), which is caused by the FIP1L1-PDGFR-alpha fusion protein. Expression of FIP1L1-PDFGR-alpha in human hematopoietic progenitors induces a myeloproliferative phenotype via activation of multiple signaling molecules, including phosphatidylinositol-3-kinase, ERK1/2, and STAT5 [11]. Imatinib has also been shown to display equally impressive therapeutic activity in eosinophilia-associated chronic myeloproliferative disorders, characterized by activating mutations of either the *PDGFR-alpha* or the *PDGFR-beta* gene by FIP1L1-PDGFR-alpha and FIP1L1-PDGFR-beta fusion proteins, respectively. The former usually results from an interstitial deletion involving chromosome 4q12, and the latter from translocations involving chromosome 5q31/33 [12]. A variant of systemic mastocytosis with eosinophilia [13] is also characterized by the expression of F1PL1-PDGFR-alpha fusion protein, and results in constitutive signaling through PDGFR-alpha. Its inhibition by treatment with Imatinib has been a successful therapeutic approach. In contrast, Imatinib is ineffective *in vitro* and *in vivo* against the mastocytosis-associated c-KIT D816V mutation [14].

NAD(P)H Dehydrogenase, Quinone 2 (NQO2)

Two recent studies have used cell extracts from the CML cell line K562 to identify binding targets of Imatinib with methods of attachment to solid support and mass spectrometry [15, 16]. Both studies identified the first non-tyrosine kinase target of Imatinib, the NAD(P)H dehydrogenase, quinone 2, also known as NQO2, a phase II detoxification enzyme which can carry out two or four electron reductions. The structural flexibility (analyzed by crystal structure at 1.75 A of a dimer of human NQ02 bound to Imatinib) that allows Imatinib to bind to NQ02 [17] has been proposed as the basis for its binding to other, more clinically relevant targets.

Discoidin Domain Receptor 1 (DDR1)

In one of the two original studies on Imatinib and NQO2 [6], the DDR1 receptor tyrosine kinase was identified as an additional Imatinib target. The inhibition of DDR1 tyrosine kinase activity by Imatinib was subsequently confirmed by Day et al. [18], which cloned and expressed human DDR1, and developed appropriate biochemical and cellular functional assays. The DDR1 inhibitory activity of Imatinib may have therapeutic implications in a number of inflammatory, fibrotic and neoplastic diseases.

vATPase

Screening in yeast identified the vacuolar proton-translocating ATPase (vATPase), an evolutionary conserved proton pump, as a novel Imatinib target. The physiological acidification of the vacuole was severely compromised following Imatinib treatment of yeast cells, an effect that was found to be dose-dependent [19]. A subsequent study from the same group [20], employing a more complex proteomics approach in yeast, confirmed these findings. Although vATPase is ubiquitously expressed in humans, its relevance for the clinical mechanism of Imatinib is presently unknown.

ABL-Related Gene (ARG)

Dysfunction of the endothelial barrier, a contributing factor of edema formation, occurs in a wide spectrum of diseases. A recent report showed that short-term treatment with Imatinib was associated with fast resolution of pulmonary edema [21]. Experimental evidence [22, 23] indicates that Imatinib exerts this effect through inhibition of ARG, a widely expressed tyrosine kinase that shares substantial sequence identity with c-ABL in the kinase domain. Although the function(s) of ARG are not well known, it is known to cooperate with c-ABL in the regulation of neurulation in the developing mouse embryo [24]. ARG inhibition prevents dysfunction of the endothelial barrier and consequently protects against vascular leakage and edema formation. Interestingly, in a systematic siRNA knock-down of the Imatinib-sensitive kinases c-ABL, ARG, PDGFR and c-KIT, only ARG knock-down had a barrier protection effect similar to that of Imatinib [23].

Gamma-Secretase-Activating Protein (GSAP)

Formation of beta-amyloid, a major hallmark of Alzheimer's disease, is catalyzed by gamma-secretase, a protease with numerous substrates. In 2010, Greengard's group [25] identified GSAP as an additional Imatinib target. They demonstrated that Imatinib lowered beta-amyloid by preventing GSAP interaction with gamma-secretase and its substrate, the amyloid precursor protein carboxy-terminal fragment (APP-CTF). Thus, GSAP can serve as a beta-amyloid lowering therapeutic target without affecting other key functions of gamma-secretase, and this suggests a potential therapeutic role of Imatinib in Alzheimer's disease.

Colony Stimulating Factor 1 Receptor (c-FMS)

In 2005, Dewar et al [26] found that Imatinib also inhibits at similar therapeutic concentrations the growth of some non-malignant hematopoietic cells, including monocyte/macrophages, through the inhibition of phosphorylation of c-FMS. Inhibition was observed at concentrations of Imatinib that are within the therapeutic dose range (IC50 = 1.42 micromolar), but its potency of inhibition was lower than what observed for c-ABL (IC50 = 0.25 micromolar), c-KIT (IC50 = 0.1 micromolar), or PDGF receptor tyrosine kinases (IC50 = 0.25 micromolar). In clinical settings, these findings caution against the possible development of significant monocytopenia where combination therapies that block multiple pathways are used, such as the association of Imatinib with interferon-alpha or cytarabine [27-29].

Besides the role of c-FMS in monocytes/macrophages, abnormal c-FMS expression correlates with adverse clinical prognosis and tumor cell invasiveness in breast and advanced epithelial ovarian carcinomas, and breast cancers producing macrophage-colony stimulating factor (M-CSF) have been implicated with promotion of bone metastases [30, 31]. Activation of c-FMS seems to stimulate tumor invasion [32, 33]. Therefore, Imatinib should be assessed for activity in diseases where abnormal c-FMS activation is implicated, including breast and ovarian cancer and inflammatory conditions, such as rheumatoid arthritis. Outside the hematopoietic system, it should be noted that c-FMS signaling plays an important role in pregnancy, affecting pre-implantation, embryo development and mammary gland development [34].

Taylor et al. [35] reported that mutation of Asp 802 of c-FMS to Val conferred Imatinib resistance. In the same study, Imatinib readily reverted the transformed phenotype of hematopoietic and fibroblast cell lines expressing c-FMS and also inhibited the growth of the Bacl.2F5 macrophage cell line, with cellular IC50 values of imatinib for c-FMS similar to those for BCR-ABL and c-KIT.

M-CSF signals are also essential for the differentiation of osteoclasts, and bone metastases of breast cancer are frequently associated with osteoclastic bone destruction. Based on these observations, Hiraga et al. [36] showed by co-immunoprecipitation that Imatinib inhibited the M-CSF-induced phosphorylation of c-FMS in osteoclast precursor cells as well as the PDGF-induced PDGFR phosphorylation in MDA-MB-231 human breast cancer cells. Imatinib also markedly reduced osteoclast formation *in vitro*. In a nude mouse model, Imatinib significantly decreased bone metastases of MDA-MB-231 breast cancer cells associated with reduced number of osteoclasts. In support of these findings, the same group reported that a specific inhibitor of c-FMS also decreased bone metastases [36], suggesting that Imatinib reduced bone metastases, at least in part, by inhibiting osteoclastic bone destruction through the blockade of c-FMS signals. At the same time, Imatinib may have a protective effect in the clinics against cancer treatment-induced bone loss.

Farnesoid X Receptor (FXR Gene)

Imatinib has also been found to modulate the FXR gene, a ligand-activated transcription factor involved in key regulation mechanisms within glucose and lipid homeostasis [37]. FXR activation and modulation of gene transcription of FXR target genes involved in glucose and lipid metabolism were proposed as biochemical consequences of Imatinib treatment. Interestingly, a case of a CML patient with type 2 diabetes who upon Imatinib treatment became insulin-independent was previously reported [38], as well as several clinical observations of diabetes remission and improved insulin sensitivity [39, 40]. Imatinib can be a starting point for anti-diabetic drug discovery with FXR-modulating activity.

Micro-RNA

Recently, Imatinib has been studied *in vitro* in the context of microRNA regulation. Yu et al. [41] reported that Imatinib markedly inhibits in human CML cells expression of miR-30a. This species of microRNA is a potent inhibitor of autophagy, acting through down-regulation of beclin 1 and ATG5 expression. Interestingly, knocking down miR-30a results in inhibition of Imatinib-induced cytotoxicity, suggesting that miR-30a and the pathways leading to autophagy may be involved in the mechanism of action of Imatinib.

Potential Pro-Malignant Activity of Imatinib

Due to the frequent expression of c-ABL, c-KIT and PDGFRs in breast cancer cells, the clinical efficacy of Imatinib has been investigated in patients with advanced and metastatic breast cancer [42, 43]. Investigating *in vitro* and in xenografts the effects of Imatinib mesylate on the human MA-11 breast carcinoma cell line, expressing both c-ABL and PDGFR-beta, Rappa et al. [44] reported that Imatinib selected cells with increased motility and aggressive behavior. Also, intraperitoneal treatment of MA-11 xenografts with Imatinib did not result in an antitumor effect, but rather increased the tumor take rate and caused the appearance of large abdominal masses in 30% of mice. Although in that study increased promoter activity driven by both Wnt and MAPK/ERK-1/2 was observed, the molecular mechanism at the basis of the pro-malignant effect of Imatinib is at present not clear. The authors hypothesized that the *in vivo* effects of Imatinib on MA-11 xenografts could be mediated, at least in part, by an immunosuppressive effect of the drug. In fact, Imatinib reportedly inhibits activation, differentiation, and proliferation of normal T lymphocytes [45], antigen presentation by dendritic cells [46], and TNF-alpha secretion [47]. Also, Cristofanilli et al. (43) reported Imatinib-mediated inhibition of interferon-gamma production by TCR-activated CD4+ T cells in patients with PDGFR-beta-expressing advanced breast cancer. Acceleration of tumor growth by Imatinib was also reported by Samoszuk et al. [48]. Growth acceleration was associated to peritumoral blood clotting. The authors proposed as a mechanism an effect of Imatinib on the tumor-infiltrating stromal mast cells. Another study [49] indicated an antagonistic effect between Imatinib and the anti-CD20 monoclonal antibody Rituximab. Thus, Imatinib reduced Rituximab-induced tumor growth inhibition in immuno-deficient mice implanted with Epstein-Barr virus-associated human B-cell lymphoma.

Conclusion

Study of the off-target effects of Imatinib have resulted in major therapeutic implications, and have suggested additional future clinical applications. The efficacy of Imatinib against multiple diseases stems from the drug ability to act against common molecular pathways and emphasizes new approaches to drug development, as cancers and diseases with varying origins and locations can respond similarly to certain drug treatments due to shared disease pathways. Additional studies are still necessary to fully elucidate the molecular mechanisms of action of Imatinib, to assess the relevance of the different secondary targets in specific diseases and to unleash its full therapeutic potential.

References

[1] Druker BJ, Talpaz M, Resta DJ, et al. Efficacy and safety of a specific inhibitor of the BCR-ABL tyrosine kinase in chronic myeloid leukemia. *N. Engl. J. Med.* 2001;344:1031-7.

[2] Gambacorti-Passerini C, Antolini L, Mahon FX, et al. Multicenter independent assessment of outcomes in chronic myeloid leukemia patients treated with imatinib. *J. Natl. Cancer Inst.*;103:553-61.

[3] Siehl J, Thiel E. C-kit, GIST, and imatinib. *Recent Results Cancer Res* 2007;176:145-51.

[4] Horak P, Wohrer A, Hassler M, Hainfellner J, Preusser M, Marosi C. Imatinib mesylate treatment of recurrent meningiomas in preselected patients: a retrospective analysis. *J. Neurooncol.*;109:323-30.

[5] Liu Y, Parry JA, Chin A, Duensing S, Duensing A. Soluble histone H2AX is induced by DNA replication stress and sensitizes cells to undergo apoptosis. *Mol. Cancer* 2008;7:61.

[6] Zhang YJ, Lu CR, Cao Y, et al. Imatinib induces H2AX phosphorylation and apoptosis in chronic myelogenous leukemia cells in vitro via caspase-3/Mst1 pathway. *Acta Pharmacol. Sin.*;33:551-7.

[7] Liu Y, Tseng M, Perdreau SA, et al. Histone H2AX is a mediator of gastrointestinal stromal tumor cell apoptosis following treatment with imatinib mesylate. *Cancer Res.* 2007;67:2685-92.

[8] Yang FC, Ingram DA, Chen S, et al. Nf1-dependent tumors require a microenvironment containing Nf1+/-- and c-kit-dependent bone marrow. *Cell* 2008;135:437-48.

[9] Hofmann UB, Kauczok-Vetter CS, Houben R, Becker JC. Overexpression of the KIT/SCF in uveal melanoma does not translate into clinical efficacy of imatinib mesylate. *Clin. Cancer Res.* 2009;15:324-9.

[10] Boucher P, Gotthardt M, Li WP, Anderson RG, Herz J. LRP: role in vascular wall integrity and protection from atherosclerosis. *Science* 2003;300:329-32.

[11] Buitenhuis M, Verhagen LP, Cools J, Coffer PJ. Molecular mechanisms underlying FIP1L1-PDGFRA-mediated myeloproliferation. *Cancer Res.* 2007;67:3759-66.

[12] Pardanani A, Ketterling RP, Brockman SR, et al. CHIC2 deletion, a surrogate for FIP1L1-PDGFRA fusion, occurs in systemic mastocytosis associated with eosinophilia and predicts response to imatinib mesylate therapy. *Blood* 2003;102:3093-6.
[13] Pardanani A, Elliott M, Reeder T, et al. Imatinib for systemic mast-cell disease. *Lancet* 2003;362:535-6.
[14] Loules G, Kalala F, Giannakoulas N, Papadakis E, Matsouka P, Speletas M. FIP1L1-PDGFRA molecular analysis in the differential diagnosis of eosinophilia. *BMC Blood* Disord. 2009;9:1.
[15] Rix U, Hantschel O, Durnberger G, et al. Chemical proteomic profiles of the BCR-ABL inhibitors imatinib, nilotinib, and dasatinib reveal novel kinase and nonkinase targets. *Blood* 2007;110:4055-63.
[16] Bantscheff M, Eberhard D, Abraham Y, et al. Quantitative chemical proteomics reveals mechanisms of action of clinical ABL kinase inhibitors. *Nat. Biotechnol.* 2007;25:1035-44.
[17] Winger JA, Hantschel O, Superti-Furga G, Kuriyan J. The structure of the leukemia drug imatinib bound to human quinone reductase 2 (NQO2). *BMC Struct. Biol.* 2009;9:7.
[18] Day E, Waters B, Spiegel K, et al. Inhibition of collagen-induced discoidin domain receptor 1 and 2 activation by imatinib, nilotinib and dasatinib. *Eur. J. Pharmacol.* 2008;599:44-53.
[19] dos Santos SC, Sa-Correia I. Genome-wide identification of genes required for yeast growth under imatinib stress: vacuolar H+-ATPase function is an important target of this anticancer drug. *OMICS* 2009;13:185-98.
[20] Dos Santos SC, Mira NP, Moreira AS, Sa-Correia I. Quantitative- and phospho-proteomic analysis of the yeast response to the tyrosine kinase inhibitor imatinib to pharmacoproteomics-guided drug line extension. *OMICS*;16:537-51.
[21] Overbeek MJ, van Nieuw Amerongen GP, Boonstra A, Smit EF, Vonk-Noordegraaf A. Possible role of imatinib in clinical pulmonary veno-occlusive disease. *Eur. Respir. J.* 2008;32:232-5.
[22] Okuda K, Weisberg E, Gilliland DG, Griffin JD. ARG tyrosine kinase activity is inhibited by STI571. *Blood* 2001;97:2440-8.
[23] Aman J, van Bezu J, Vogel SM, et al. Imatinib: A novel candidate for treatment of permeability edema. *American Journal of Respiratory and Critical Care Medicine* 2012;185:A3661.
[24] Koleske AJ, Gifford AM, Scott ML, et al. Essential roles for the Abl and Arg tyrosine kinases in neurulation. *Neuron* 1998;21:1259-72.
[25] He G, Luo W, Li P, et al. Gamma-secretase activating protein is a therapeutic target for Alzheimer's disease. *Nature;*467:95-8.
[26] Dewar AL, Cambareri AC, Zannettino AC, et al. Macrophage colony-stimulating factor receptor c-fms is a novel target of imatinib. *Blood* 2005;105:3127-32.
[27] Gardembas M, Rousselot P, Tulliez M, et al. Results of a prospective phase 2 study combining imatinib mesylate and cytarabine for the treatment of Philadelphia-positive patients with chronic myelogenous leukemia in chronic phase. *Blood* 2003;102:4298-305.
[28] Kantarjian HM, O'Brien S, Cortes J, et al. Imatinib mesylate therapy improves survival in patients with newly diagnosed Philadelphia chromosome-positive chronic

myelogenous leukemia in the chronic phase: comparison with historic data. *Cancer* 2003;98:2636-42.
[29] Wassmann B, Scheuring U, Pfeifer H, et al. Efficacy and safety of imatinib mesylate (Glivec) in combination with interferon-alpha (IFN-alpha) in Philadelphia chromosome-positive acute lymphoblastic leukemia (Ph+ALL). *Leukemia* 2003;17:1919-24.
[30] Toy EP, Chambers JT, Kacinski BM, Flick MB, Chambers SK. The activated macrophage colony-stimulating factor (CSF-1) receptor as a predictor of poor outcome in advanced epithelial ovarian carcinoma. *Gynecol. Oncol.* 2001;80:194-200.
[31] Sapi E. The role of CSF-1 in normal physiology of mammary gland and breast cancer: an update. *Exp. Biol. Med.* (Maywood) 2004;229:1-11.
[32] Kacinski BM. CSF-1 and its receptor in breast carcinomas and neoplasms of the female reproductive tract. *Mol. Reprod. Dev.* 1997;46:71-4.
[33] Sapi E, Kacinski BM. The role of CSF-1 in normal and neoplastic breast physiology. *Proc. Soc. Exp. Biol. Med.* 1999;220:1-8.
[34] Pollard JW. Role of colony-stimulating factor-1 in reproduction and development. *Mol. Reprod. Dev.* 1997;46:54-60; discussion -1.
[35] Taylor JR, Brownlow N, Domin J, Dibb NJ. FMS receptor for M-CSF (CSF-1) is sensitive to the kinase inhibitor imatinib and mutation of Asp-802 to Val confers resistance. *Oncogene* 2006;25:147-51.
[36] Hiraga T, Nakamura H. Imatinib mesylate suppresses bone metastases of breast cancer by inhibiting osteoclasts through the blockade of c-Fms signals. *Int. J. Cancer* 2009;124:215-22.
[37] Steri R, Achenbach J, Steinhilber D, Schubert-Zsilavecz M, Proschak E. Investigation of imatinib and other approved drugs as starting points for antidiabetic drug discovery with FXR modulating activity. *Biochem. Pharmacol.*;83:1674-81.
[38] Veneri D, Franchini M, Bonora E. Imatinib and regression of type 2 diabetes. N. *Engl. J. Med.* 2005;352:1049-50.
[39] Breccia M, Muscaritoli M, Aversa Z, Mandelli F, Alimena G. Imatinib mesylate may improve fasting blood glucose in diabetic Ph+ chronic myelogenous leukemia patients responsive to treatment. *J. Clin. Oncol.* 2004;22:4653-5.
[40] Tsapas A, Vlachaki E, Sarigianni M, Klonizakis F, Paletas K. Restoration of insulin sensitivity following treatment with imatinib mesylate (Gleevec) in non-diabetic patients with chronic myelogenic leukemia (CML). *Leuk. Res.* 2008;32:674-5.
[41] Yu Y, Yang L, Zhao M, et al. Targeting microRNA-30a-mediated autophagy enhances imatinib activity against human chronic myeloid leukemia cells. *Leukemia*;26:1752-60.
[42] Chew HK, Barlow WE, Albain K, et al. A phase II study of imatinib mesylate and capecitabine in metastatic breast cancer: Southwest Oncology Group Study 0338. *Clin. Breast Cancer* 2008;8:511-5.
[43] Cristofanilli M, Morandi P, Krishnamurthy S, et al. Imatinib mesylate (Gleevec) in advanced breast cancer-expressing C-Kit or PDGFR-beta: clinical activity and biological correlations. *Ann. Oncol.* 2008;19:1713-9.
[44] Rappa G, Anzanello F, Lorico A. Imatinib mesylate enhances the malignant behavior of human breast carcinoma cells. *Cancer Chemother Pharmacol* 2011;67:919-26.
[45] Cwynarski K, Laylor R, Macchiarulo E, et al. Imatinib inhibits the activation and proliferation of normal T lymphocytes in vitro. *Leukemia* 2004;18:1332-9.

[46] Seggewiss R, Price DA, Purbhoo MA. Immunomodulatory effects of imatinib and second-generation tyrosine kinase inhibitors on T cells and dendritic cells: an update. *Cytotherapy* 2008;10:633-41.

[47] Wolf AM, Wolf D, Rumpold H, et al. The kinase inhibitor imatinib mesylate inhibits TNF-{alpha} production in vitro and prevents TNF-dependent acute hepatic inflammation. *Proc. Natl. Acad. Sci. USA* 2005;102:13622-7.

[48] Samoszuk M, Corwin MA. Acceleration of tumor growth and peri-tumoral blood clotting by imatinib mesylate (Gleevec). *Int. J. Cancer* 2003;106:647-52.

[49] Nemati F, Mathiot C, Grandjean I, et al. Imatinib mesylate reduces rituximab-induced tumor-growth inhibition in vivo on Epstein-Barr virus-associated human B-cell lymphoma. *Anticancer Drugs* 2007;18:1029-37.

In: Imatinib
Editors: Mojtaba Akhtari and Ihab Elhemaidi
ISBN: 978-1-62808-297-5

Chapter 10

Activity of Imatinib Mesylate in Metastatic Melanoma

Paolo Savoia* and Paolo Fava
Department of Biomedical Sciences and Human Oncology, Section of Dermatology, University of Turin, Torino, Italia

Abstract

KIT, a type III transmembrane receptor tyrosine kinase, plays a central role in cancer cell proliferation, invasion and metastases, through the activation of several signalling pathways. In melanocytes, KIT function is critical for the normal development and in melanoma KIT play a predominant role as tumour suppressor. KIT gene alterations, such as activating mutations or increased copy number, are relatively commonly demonstrated in melanomas arising in acral, mucosal and chronically sun-damaged sites. Over 21 different mutations of the KIT gene have been found; however, similar to GIST, the majority of these mutations occur within the juxtamembrane authoinhibitory region encoded by exon 11. Some studies assessed that KIT could impact melanoma progression, suggesting that KIT-target therapies would be useful in advanced stage of disease. However, not all KIT mutations give the same responses to Imatinib. Despite the fact that L576P and K642E amino acid substitutions, that are the most common KIT alterations in melanomas, are more sensitive to KIT inhibitors, three phase 2 studies did not demonstrated clinical activity of Imatinib in treatment of unselected metastatic melanoma patients. In fact, only a subset of melanomas with genetic alteration of Kit responds to treatment, and genetic selection of KIT aberrations is a prerequisite for Imatinib-based therapy in metastatic melanoma In this chapter are extensively explained the most recent literature data about the role of Imatinib in the treatment of metastatic melanoma; the mechanisms of treatment resistance and how to treat Imatinib-resistant patients are also discussed.

* Corresponding author: Tel. 011/6335816, Fax 011/6335034, Email: paola.savoia@unito.it.

Introduction

KIT, a type III transmembrane receptor tyrosine kinase, plays a central role in cancer cell proliferation, invasion and metastases, through the activation of several signalling pathways. In melanocytes, KIT function is critical for the normal development and, in melanoma, it plays a predominant role as tumour suppressor.

KIT gene alterations, as activating mutations or increased copy number, are relatively commonly demonstrated in melanomas arising in acral, mucosal and chronically sun-damaged sites. Over 21 different mutations of the KIT gene have been found; similar to GIST, the majority of these mutations occur within the juxtamembrane authoinhibitory region encoded by exon 11. Some studies assessed that KIT could impact melanoma progression, suggesting that KIT-target therapies would be useful in advanced stage of disease. However, not all KIT mutations give the same responses to Imatinib. Despite the fact that L576P and K642E amino acid substitutions, that are the most common KIT alterations in melanomas, are more sensitive to KIT inhibitors, three phase 2 studies did not demonstrated clinical activity of Imatinib in treatment of unselected metastatic melanoma patients. In fact, only a subset of melanomas with genetic alteration of KIT responds to treatment, and genetic selection of KIT aberrations is a prerequisite for Imatinib-based therapy in metastatic melanoma.

In this chapter are extensively explained the most recent literature data about the role of Imatinib in the treatment of metastatic melanoma; the mechanisms of treatment resistance and how to treat Imatinib-resistant patients are also discussed.

Molecular Basis

The importance of KIT in normal melanocyte development is well characterized (Hou 2000, Wehrle-Haller 2003, Alexeev 2006). KIT encodes a type III transmembrane receptor tyrosine kinase in which the juxtamembrane domain plays an autoinhibitory role, preventing KIT activation in absence of ligand. Binding of KIT's ligand to the extracellular domain causes the KIT receptor to dimerize, resulting in autophosphorylation of the intracellular tyrosine kinase domains. Once activated, the tyrosine kinase domains initiate signalling in a variety of downstream pathways including the MAPK/MEK, phosphatidylinositol, 3-OH kinase/AKT, JAK/signal transducers and activators of transcription pathways.

KIT function is critical in normal melanocyte development (Natali 1992, Montoni 1997); a study by Huang et al (1996) showed that the highly metastatic melanoma cell line A375SM had reduced ability to form metastases and increased apoptotic sensitivity after transfection with the KIT gene. Immunohistochemical studies showed that loss of the gene product of KIT correlated with transformation, invasion, and metastasis. (Natali 1992). Moreover, loss of KIT expression is observed with progression of disease from superficial to invasive to metastatic stages, suggesting that KIT possesses tumour suppressive functions (Lassam 1992, Natali 1992, Zakut 1993, Huang 1996, Montoni 1997).

Even if the most frequent mutations in cutaneous melanoma involve BRAF sequences, melanomas arising from acral, mucosal, or skin that has suffered chronic sun damage, have most frequently amplifications or activating mutations of c-KIT (Curtin 2005; Curtin 2006, Beadling 2008, Postow 2012).

Table 1. Percentual distribution of melanoma mutations in some literature series

	BRAF			GNAQ			KIT			NRAS			Wildtype		
All melanomas	45[1]	-	56[3]	4[1]	-	-	3[1]	-	0[3]	2[1]	-	-	28[1]	-	-
Acral	23[1]	23[2]	21[3]	1[1]	1[2]	-	24[1]	38[2]	36[3]	16[1]	15[2]	-	36[1]	-	-
Chronical sun-damaged skin	22[1]	22[2]	6[3]	0[1]	0[2]	-	19[1]	32[2]	28[3]	0[1]	0[2]	-	59[1]	-	-
Mucosal	9[1]	9[2]	3[3]	0[1]	0[2]	-	25[1]	43[2]	39[3]	11[1]	12[2]	-	55[1]	-	-

[1]Postow; [2]Carvajal; [3]Curtin

In Asia, acral and mucosal melanoma account for about 70% of all melanomas; as a consequence c-KIT mutations are the most frequent genetic abnormality in Asian population (Li 2010).

Over 21 different mutations of the KIT gene have been found, mainly in exons 9, 11, 13, 17 and 18.1,6–21. Most mutations occur in the juxtamembrane region of exon 11 (L576P) and exon 13 (K642E). The spectrum of mutations observed in melanomas reflects those reported in gastrointestinal stromal tumours (GIST); in particular, many of the KIT mutations affect the exon 11, that encode for the juxtamembrane inhibitory domain (Lennartsson 1999, Heinrich 2003).

Clinical Experience

Clinical studies with Imatinib have demonstrated stable and responding disease rates ranging from 75 to 90% in advanced GIST and CML; however, the percentage of melanoma patients in which Imatinib is effective is still debated (Hodi 2008). In fact, even if many studies gave encouraging results (Lutzky 2008, Kim 2008, Satzger 2010, Yamaguchi 2010, Arifi 2011), there are several cases, including acro-lentiginous and mucosal melanoma, that failed Imatinib therapy after an initial response.

In 2008, Imatinib was used as single-agent in a Phase II trial on 21 metastatic melanoma patients that expressed at least one protein tyrosine kinase (Kim 2008). Imatinib was administered orally at a dose of 400 mg twice a day, until there was evidences of disease progression or unacceptable toxicity. Among the 21 patients treated, only 4 (20%) had a disease stabilization, which lasted less than 13 week and one patient (5%) had a durable partial response (12.8 months). More in details, this patient had a near complete response by fluorodeoxyglucose-positron emission tomography (FDG-PET)/computed tomography (CT) and greater than 50% tumor reduction after 4 weeks of imatinib therapy, without significant treatment-related toxicity.

However, the majority of patients experienced an early progression of the disease, such as reported also in other previous clinical trials. In 2005, Ugurel showed that there was no clinical response among 16 patients treated with Imatinb; this lack of efficacy was also observed in another clinical trial, in which Imatinib was administered according the same schedule, with high-grade systemic side-effects and without appreciable clinical results (Wyman 2006).

Despite these few encouraging initial results, multiple studies since then have demonstrated the effectiveness of Imatinib in selected groups of melanoma patients with KIT alterations (Carvajal 2011, Guo 2011). After a careful patient accrual, Guo et al. demonstrated significant benefits of Imatinib treatment in a group of stage IV melanoma patients with either KIT mutations and/or KIT amplification. This open-label/single arm study enrolled 43 patients. Imatinib 400 mg/day was given to all participants with dose escalation to 800 mg/day allowed in those who experienced disease progression. The median progression-free survival (PFS) was 3.5 months whereas the 6-month PFS was 36.6% (Korn 2008). Partial response (PR), which was one of the secondary end points, was observed in 10 patients (23.3%). Similarly, Carvajal et al. were able to demonstrate significant durable responses of greater than 1 year in 4 of 25 patients who harbored the KIT mutation and/or amplification; two other patients from this group experienced a complete response. Both studies confirmed that an accurate selection of melanoma patients before the treatment with Imatinib is mandatory in order to increase the rate of clinical response. This observation was underlined also by a recent study published by Schoenewolf et al, who demonstrated the presence of kit mutation in *ex vivo* lines from Imatinib responder patients (Schoenewolf 2011).

Other data confirmed that mutations in exon 11 and 13 were most predictive of response to Imatinib whereas mutations in exons 9, 17 and 18 did not. Specifically, Carvajal et al. showed that responder patients harbored either the L576P or K642E mutations in exon 11 and 13, respectively. Conversely, they putted into the light that non-responders patients harbored specific KIT mutations known to confer Imatinib resistance also in GIST, such as D820Y/N822K and A829P in exons 17 and 18, respectively.

It is noteworthy that clinical results were obtained even with a dose of Imatinib lower than the standard. Yamaguchi et al (2010), described a case of a KIT mutation-positive metastatic melanoma that markedly regressed within 2 weeks of treatment with Imatinib mesylate. Treatment was initially started at 400 mg/day, but rapidly reduced to 200 mg/day as a consequence of grade 2 gastro-intestinal and skin toxicities. Depsite this dose reduction, clinical response was observed and maintained after a follow up of 4 months.

It is interesting to note that some recent experimental data *in vivo* on mice melanoma cell demonstrated that Imatinib can enhance dacarbazine uptake and activity. Further data are needed to evaluate if this synergistic activity could be useful also in human (Ogawa 2008).

As expected from the experience learned in others fields of applications, Imatinib toxicity resulted dose related. The most common side effects were haematological, intestinal and dermatological. In the majority of cases the observed toxicities were grade 1-2, even if in larger studies (Ugurel, 2005), severe toxicity leading to dose modification occurred in 39% of patients. However, also in grade 3 or 4 reactions, all toxicity rapidly resolved after drug suspension.

Imatinib Resistance and Further Perspectives

No data are available about Imatinib resistance in melanoma. However, Imatinib-resistant GIST has been extensively studied; in fact, some patients after a period of initial response or stable disease develop resistance to the drug, within 12-36 months of treatment (Vassos 2011). Imatinib resistance in GIST is commonly classified into two categories: primary and secondary resistance (Tran 2012). Primary resistance is observed in approximately 14% of GIST patients and is defined by KIT-mutated GISTs not responding to Imatinib on initial exposure. Secondary resistance develops in 40% to 50% of patients after an initial tumor response to Imatinib. The mechanism of primary resistance could be explained by activation of the AKT/mTOR signalling pathways, as suggested by Sapi et al (2011). They also underlined that the inhibition of the mTOR signalling pathway could represent a further therapeutic target. A role for oncogenic pathway involving the insulin-like growth factor 1 receptor (IGF-1R) has also postulated: IGF-1R is a tyrosine kinase protein involved in the regulation of cellular proliferation that is significantly increased in GISTs without the KIT or PDGFR mutation (Pantaleo 2010).

The mechanisms responsible for the secondary resistance were found to be very heterogeneous and include functional resistance in wild-type *c-Kit*, presence of secondary mutations, target gene amplification and activation of other alternative kinases, that parallels the finding of cytoarchitectural and immunophenotypic changes observed in GIST tumours after Imatinib treatment (Vassos, 2011).

Data emerging from recent literature studies suggest that various secondary KIT or PDGFRA mutations exist in more than 50% of resistant patients. In this subgroup of patients, other second generation KIT inhibitors, such as Sunitinib, Sorafenib, Nilotinib, Dasatinib and Masanitib should be tested. Woodman et al. recently demonstrated the potential utility of dasatinib in metastatic melanoma with KIT mutation (2009) in two patients affected by metastatic melanoma with L576P-specific KIT mutation. On the contrary, a recent phase II study by Kluger et al. (2011) using dasatinib in 39 unselected patients with metastatic melanoma did not achieve the end points of 30% response rate or 6-month PFS.

Moreover, mutations in the ATP-binding domain (such as T670I and V654A) are a potential target for another second generation KIT inhibitor Nilotinib, even if these mutations in the activation loop are difficult to overcome pharmacologically.

In 2010, a phase III randomized trial with Nilotinib versus DTIC was started; unfortunately, only few patients met the inclusion criteria and the study was converted in a single-arm phase II trial with Nilotinib alone (Kluger 2011).

Data about melanoma patients are to date too scanty; however, the experience on GIST patients suggests a potential role of sequencing therapy with Nilotinib in patients progressed during imatinib treatment.

Recently, histone deacetylase inhibitors (HDACi) were used to targeting secondary imatinib resistance in GIST. The antitumor activity seems to be mediated by the suppression of deacylation of its chaperone protein, heat-shock protein 90 (HSP90) that results in the inactivation of the oncogenic signalling cascade (Muhlenberg 2009)

Also mammalian target of Rapamicin (mTOR) inhibitor as everolimus has been recently used in a Imatinib-resistant patient that achieved a partial response. This observation suggests a potential role of mTOR as a mediator of acquired Imatinib resistance in melanoma (Si 2012).

Conclusion

Imatinib inhibitor may represent a useful tool in the treatment of some selected categories of melanoma patients. The right selection of these subpopulations of patients whose tumors are driven by an activating mutation of c-kit is mandatory. Another crucial challenge will be the development of additional small molecules that will overcome primary and secondary resistances.

References

Alexeev, V; Yoon, K. Distinctive role of the cKit receptor tyrosine kinase signaling in mammalian melanocytes. *J Invest Dermatol.* 2006; 126, 1102-1110.

Arifi, S; Tazi, EM; El Mesbahi, O; Errihani, H. Activity of Imatinib Mesylate in Metastatic Anorectal Melanoma, A Case Report. *J Gastrointest Canc*, 2011; 11, 1-3.

Beadling, C; Jacobson-Dunlop, E; Hodi, FS; et al. KIT gene mutations and copy number in melanoma subtypes. *Clin Cancer Res.* 2008; 14, 6821- 6828.

Carvajal, RD; Antonescu, CR; Wolchok, JD; et al. KIT as a therapeutic target in metastatic melanoma. *JAMA*, 2011; 305, 2327-2334.

Curtin, JA; Fridlyand, J; Kageshita, T; et al. Distinct sets of genetic alterations in melanoma. *N Engl J Med.* 2005; 353, 2135-2147.

Curtin, JA; Busam, K; Pinkel, D; et al. Somatic activation of KIT in distinct subtypes of melanoma. *J Clin Oncol.* 2006; 24, 4340- 4346.

Guo, J; Si, L; Kong, Y; et al. Phase II, open-label, single-arm trial of imatinib mesylate in patients with metastatic melanoma harboring c-kit mutation or amplification. *J Clin Oncol*, 2011; 29, 2904-2909.

Heinrich, MC; Corless, CL; Demetri, GD; et al. Kinase mutations and imatinib response in patients with metastatic gastrointestinal stromal tumor. *J Clin Oncol.* 2003; 21, 4342-4349.

Hodi, FS; Friedlander, P; Corless, CL; et al. Major response to imatinib mesylate in KIT-mutated melanoma. *J Clin Oncol*, 2008; 26, 2046–2051.

Hou, L; Panthier, JJ; Arnheiter, H. Signaling and transcriptional regulation in the neural crest-derived melanocyte lineage, interactions between KIT and MITF. *Development.* 2000; 127, 5379-5389.

Huang, S; Luca, M; Gutman, M; et al. Enforced c-KIT expression renders highly metastatic human melanoma cells susceptible to stem cell factor-induced apoptosis and inhibits their tumorigenic and metastatic potential. *Oncogene.* 1996; 13, 2339-2347.

Kim, KB; Eton, O; Davis, DW; Frazier, ML; et al. Phase II trial of imatinib mesylate in patients with metastatic melanoma. *Br J Cancer.* 2008; 99, 734-740.

Kluger, HM; Dudek, AZ; McCann, C; et al. A phase 2 trial of dasatinib in advanced melanoma. *Cancer.* 2011; 15, 2202-2208.

Korn, EL; Liu, PY; Lee, SJ; et al. Meta-analysis of phase II cooperative group trials in metastatic stage IV melanoma to determine progression-free and overall survival benchmarks for future phase II trials. *J Clin Oncol*, 2008; 26, 527-534.

Lassam, N; Bickford, S. Loss of c-kit expression in cultured melanoma cells. *Oncogene.* 1992; 7, 51-56.

Lennartsson, J; Blume-Jensen, P; Hermanson, M; et al. Phosphorylation of Shc by Src family kinases is necessary for stem cell factor receptor/c-kit mediated activation of the Ras/MAP kinase pathway and c-fos induction. *Oncogene.* 1999; 18, 5546-5553.

Li, SM; Guo, J; Chi, ZH; et al, Melanoma in China, A prognostic study of 522 cases. *J Clin Oncol*, 28, 2010.

Lutzky, J; Bauer, J; Bastian, BC. Dose-dependent, complete response to imatinib of a metastatic mucosal melanoma with a K642E KIT mutation. *Pigment Cell Melanoma Res*, 2008; 21, 492–493.

Montone, KT; van Belle, P; Elenitsas, R; Elder, DE. Proto-oncogene c-kit expression in malignant melanoma, protein loss with tumor progression. *Mod Pathol*. 1997; 10, 939-944.

Muhlenberg, T; Zhang, Y; Wagner, AJ; et al. Inhibitors of Deacetylases suppressoncogenic KIT gastrointestinal stromal tumors signaling, acetylate HSP90, and induce apoptosis in gastrointestinal stromal tumors. *Cancer Res*, 2009; 69, 6941-6950.

Natali, PG; Nicotra, MR; Winkler, AB; et al. Progression of human cutaneous melanoma is associated with loss of expression of ckit proto-oncogene receptor. *Int J Cancer*. 1992; 52, 197-201.

Ogawa, Y; Kawamura, T; Furuhashi, M; Tsukamoto, K; Shimada, S. Improving chemotherapeutic drug penetration in melanoma by imatinib mesylate. *Journal of Dermatological Science*, 2008; 51, 190—199.

Pantaleo, MA; Astolfi, A; Nannini, M; et al. The emerging role of insulin-like growth factor 1 receptor (IGF1r) in gastrointestinal stromal tumors (GISTs). *J Transl Med*, 2010; 8, 117.

Postow, M; Carvajal, M. Therapeutic Implications of KIT in Melanoma. *The Cancer Journal & Volume*, 2012; 18, 37-142

Sapi, Z; Fule, T; Hajdu, M; et al. The activated targets of mTOR signalling pathway are characteristic for PDGFRA mutant and wild-type rather than KIT mutant GISTs. *Diagn Mol Pathol*, 2011; 20, 22-33.

Satzger, I; Kuttler, U; Volker, B; et al. Anal mucosal melanoma with KIT-activating mutation and response to imatinib therapy – case report and review of the literature. *Dermatology*, 2010; 220, 77–81.

Schoenewolf, NL; Urosevic-Maiwald, M; Dummer, R. Tumour heterogeneity of mucosal melanomas during treatment with imatinib. *Br J Dermatol*, 2011; 165, 419–424.

Si, L; Xu, X; Kong, Y; et al. Major response to everolimus in melanoma with acquired imatinib resistance. *J Clin Oncol*. 2012; 30, 37-40.

Tran, A; Tawbi, HA. A potential role for nilotinib in KIT-mutated melanoma. *Expert Opin. Investig. Drugs*, 2012; 21, 861-869.

Ugurel, S; Hildebrand, R; Zimpfer, A; La Rosee, P; et al Lack of clinical efficacy of imatinib in metastatic melanoma. *Br J Cancer*, 2005; 92, 1398-1405.

Vassos, N; Agaimy, A; Schlabrakowski, A; Hohenberger, W; Schneider-Stock, R; Croner, RS. An unusual and potentially misleading phenotypic change in a primary gastrointestinal stromal tumour (GIST) under imatinib mesylate therapy. *Virchows Arch*, 2011; 458, 363–369.

Wehrle-Haller, B. The role of Kit-ligand in melanocyte development and epidermal homeostasis. *Pigment Cell Res*. 2003; 16, 287-296.

Woodman, SE; Trent, JD; Stemke-Hale K; et al. Activity of Dasatinib Against L576P KIT Mutant Melanoma, Molecular, Cellular and Clinical Correlates. *Mol Cancer Ther*. 2009; 8, 2079–2085.

Wyman, K; Atkins, MB; Prieto, V; Eton, O; et al. Multicenter phase II trial of high-dose imatinib mesylate in metastatic melanoma, significant toxicity with no clinical efficacy. *Cancer*, 2006; 106, 2005-2011.

Yamaguchi, M; Harada, K; Ando, N; Kawamura, T; Shibagaki, N; Shimada, S. Marked response to imatinib mesylate in metastatic acral lentiginous melanoma on the thumb. *Clinical and Experimental Dermatology*, 2010; 36, 174–177.

Zakut, R; Perlis, R; Eliyahu, S; et al. KIT ligand (mast cell growth factor) inhibits the growth of KIT expressing melanoma cells. *Oncogene*. 1993; 8, 2221-2229.

In: Imatinib
Editors: Mojtaba Akhtari and Ihab Elhemaidi

ISBN: 978-1-62808-297-5

Chapter 11

Imatinib Mesylate for Advanced Melanoma Harboring C-KIT Mutations: New Treatment Selection?

Jun Guo
Department of Melanoma and Renal Cancer,
Peking University Cancer Hospital and Institute, Peking, China

Abstract

Malignant melanoma is the most frequent cause of mortality in skin cancer. Unlike those Caucasian populations, mucosal and acral melanomas account for approximately 65% of all melanomas in Chinese populations. C-KIT mutations are more common in mucosal and acral melanomas, which can also be accompanied by an increase in c-KIT copy numbers. As a potent inhibitor targeting Abl as well as c-KIT, imatinib played an important role in treatment of metastatic melanoma harboring c-KIT mutations or amplifications. In a phase II trial by Guo and colleagues, in which all paients harbored c-KIT mutations or amplifications, there was a 54% disease control rate with imatinib, the results of this trial showed imatinib may increase the overall PFS rate, the overall RR, and the OS in the selected patients with melanoma. Most adverse events were mild to moderate and well controlled. Another phase II trial by Carvajal demonstrated similar results as well. These results demonstrated that imatinib is a promising agent in selected patents of melanomas with genetic alterations of C-KIT. However, these data need to be confirmed by phase III trial or meta-analyses.

Malignant melanoma causes the most deaths in skin cancer. Up to the end of 2010, the incidence of melanoma in Beijing (China) was 8.9 per 100 thousand, which was much lower when compared with many western countries (such as USA, Australia). Although we don't have the precise value of melanoma incidence in China, the number of newly diagnosed cases annually was not small due to the large population in our country. Low incidence but high death rates are epidemiological characteristics of melanoma in China. Therefore, attention on melanoma is urgent needed.

Primary melanoma are differentiated into four subtypes depending on sun exposure and localization: acral melanoma (sun-protected skin such as the palms, soles, or subungual sites), mucosal melanoma, melanoma on chronically sun-damaged skin (skin showing evidence of chronic sun-induced damage evidenced by marked solar elastosis), and melanoma arising from skin without signs of chronic sun damage (non-CSD melanomas) [1]. The different body site distribution of primary MM is related to ethnic background. Mucosal and acral melanomas account for approximately 65% of all melanomas in Chinese populations, whereas in those Caucasian populations, the main location is trunk and legs [2, 3].

KIT Mutation and Expression Characteristics and Ethnic Differences

Molecular profiling of melanoma is found to be associated with subgroups of melanoma. C-KIT mutations and/or an increase in c-KIT copy numbers are more common in mucosal, acral and CSD melanomas, however, BRAF mutations are highly prevalent in non-CSD melanomas [1,4]. Curtin examined 102 primary melanomas and found mutations and/or copy number increases of KIT in 39% of mucosal melanomas, 36% of acral melanomas, and 28% of melanomas on chronically sun-damaged skin, no KIT mutation was found in melanomas on non chronically sun-damaged skin [1]. Beadling et al. also reported that KIT mutations were present in 23% of acral melanomas, 15.6% of mucosal melanomas, 7.7% of conjunctival melanomas, 1.7% of cutaneous melanomas, and 0% of choroidal melanomas in a cohort of 189 melanomas [5].

In our Chinese study, 502 patients were examined, the overall incidence of somatic mutations within the KIT gene was 10.8% (54/502), and all subtypes of melanoma contained KIT mutations. The frequency of KIT mutations in the acral, mucosal and CSD melanoma subgroups were 11.9% (23/193), 9.6% (16/167), and 20.7% (6/29), respectively [6]. To our knowledge this is the largest study ever performed of the KIT mutation. Ashida from Japan reported the frequency of KIT mutations in a Japanese cohort, which mainly consisted of metastatic acral melanomas, was 17% [7]. These Asian data suggested that although acral and mucosal melanoma were more prevalent in Asian population, the frequency of KIT mutations seems lower than the Caucasian patients. The reason is unclear, perhaps because the different geographic patient populations have a diverse KIT mutation status in acral and mucosal melanomas; or the Asian cohorts tested more metastatic lesions, since Shen has revealed that c-KIT expression tends to be diminished in metastatic lesions [8]. The L576P KIT mutation located at the c-terminus of KIT exon 11and K642E on exon 13 are reported to be the most common KIT mutation to date in melanoma (~30–40% of mutations) [5]. The Chinese data also showed the most frequent KIT mutations were L576P (9 cases) and K642E (5 cases), and for the first time, they declaimed that KIT mutations and genetic aberrations (mutation plus amplification) of KIT adversely impact survival [6].

KIT encodes a type III transmembrane receptor tyrosine kinase, also known as CD117, which is a cell surface receptor consisting of an extracellular domain, a transmembrane domain (coded by exon 10), and a cytoplasmic domain consisting of a juxtamembrane domain (coded by exon 11) and 2 intracellular tyrosine kinase domains (coded by exons 12-21 [9,10].C-KIT protein expression of CD117 can be detected in the majority of mucosal melanomas (up to 91% [11]), but also in a high percentage of cutaneous melanomas, up to 84% [12,13]. The association between CD117 protein expression and c-kit mutations in melanomas was studied in many different studies. Satzger et a found that 8 of the 9 anorectal melanomas were positive for CD117 expression, but only 3 showed strong expression, and 1 of the 3 tumors contained the L576P c-kit mutation [11]. Antonescu et al reported that 23% of melanomas showed a diffuse and strong reactivity to the antibody of CD117, and the 3 cases with L576P mutations were included in this assessment [14]. Kong et al further studied 502 melanoma patients, Among the 54 cases with a KIT mutation, 24 cases (44.4%) were positive for CD117, which was not significantly different to those (7.4% and 39.6% respectively) detected in the overall population. Moreover, they found that 68.8% (11/16) of mucosal melanomas with KIT mutations were positive for CD117, which, however, was not significantly higher than the staining seen in acral melanomas (34.8%), CSD melanomas (16.7%), non-CSD melanomas (60.0%), or of melanomas of unknown primary (25.0%; P=0.11) [6]. Ni et al examined 40 cases of anorectal melanoma, 16 melanomas showed diffuse and strong expression and 1 melanoma had weak and focal reactivity. Three tumors harboring c-kit mutation had diffuse and strong expression of CD117. One contained an L576P mutation, whereas another contained double mutated loci with G562V and E583V, and the third contained a W557R mutation [15]. All these study results indicated that CD117 protein expression did not correlate with the mutation status. The results were consistent with those of Curtin et al [1]. They observed the increased expression of CD117 in 33% of melanomas without detectable c-kit mutations or copy number increases. In contrast, in the Antonescu et al study, the 3 c-kit mutation tumors were strongly immunopositive for CD117. They reported that there was a higher expression of CD117 in anorectal melanomas harboring a potentially activating c-kit mutation when compared with tumors without c-kit mutations [14].

Potential Mechanism for Imatinib Targets Melanoma

Imatinib mesylate (Gleevec, formerly STI571), is a selective inhibitor, targeting ABL as well as c-KIT and the platelet-derived growth factor receptor. It was originally developed by Novartis Pharmaceuticals as a specific inhibitor of the BCR-ABL tyrosine kinase, which arises from an acquired t(9;22) genetic translocation (Philadelphia chromosome) that causes chronic myelogenous leukemia. [16]. Gastrointestinal stromal tumors often express mutated forms of c-KIT, and patients with these tumors were also found to respond to imatinib mesylate [17]. When imatinib mesylate was found effective in patients with the hypereosinophilic syndrome [18], investigation into the genetic basis of this disease revealed that many of these patients harbor a chromosomal deletion that gives rise to an oncogenic fusion protein (FIP1L1-PDGFRA) involving the PDGF receptor [19]. Imatinib mesylate is thus now considered an effective agent for many malignancies characterized by aberrant protein tyrosine kinase(PTK) signaling via ABL, c-KIT, and PDGF receptor.

Given suggestions of KIT's function as a targetable oncogene in GIST, initial hypotheses of imatinib as an anti-tumor agent in melanoma were reevaluated. There are several reasons to think that this drug may have therapeutic potential in melanoma. First, it is known that PTK signaling is critical for sustaining melanocyte proliferation in vitro and for migration of melanocytic cells in vivo [20]. In addition, overexpression of some PTK receptor ligands such as hepatocyte growth factor is associated with increased susceptibility to melanoma in mice

[21]. All three known targets of imatinib mesylate (ABL, c-KIT, PDGF receptor) are generally expressed in melanoma.

Subsequent studies evaluated the sensitivity melanoma cell lines to imatinib in vivo and in vitro. Pereira et al found that cells that were directly exposed imatinib mesylate showed a decrease in proliferation for five human uveal melanoma cell lines [22]. A report on murine B16F10 melanoma cells injected into C57B16 mice revealed the growth of primary melanoma tumors was potently suppressed by systemic Gleevec therapy. Tumor growth was inhibited by 77% at a dose of 0.75 mg five times weekly as compared with control mice treated with saline alone [23]. In vitro studies, Jiang reported cell lines treated with imatinib showed substantial anti-proliferative activity in the KIT-mutant M6 but not in the KIT wild-type mucosal melanomas [24]. Based on these preclinical studies, imatinib was led to the treatment of metastatic melanoma subsequently.

Clinical Trials Lead to an Effective Treatment Option

Previously, some case reports also showed imatinib had remarkable efficacy on KIT mutated melenomas [25, 26]. But initial phase II trials testing imatinib in genetically unselected patients with metastatic melanoma got disappointing results [27, 28, 29]. For the study of 16 cases, only two patients (12%) displayed the characteristics of high-KIT–aberration tumors (one acral melanoma, one mucosal melanoma), whereas 13 patients (81%) belonged to the group of low-KIT–aberration (ie, 11 melanomas of the trunk or extremities without chronic sun damage, four melanomas of unknown primary); one patient with a primary melanoma of the eye [27]. The Ugurel's trial didn't display the characteristics of primary sites of the enrolled patients. In the Eton's trial, patients were required to express one of the imatinib target proteins by immunohistochemistry [28]. Of the 21 patients treated with imatinib, 16 had disease progression by 6 weeks and another 4 within 12 weeks. However, 1 patient with strong c-KIT expression in greater than 75% of cells had a near-complete response for more than a year. The patient had the c-KIT RNA of his melanoma sequenced, which revealed a deletion in codon 715 [29].

As disappointing as the results of these studies were, they were still the first attempt of "targeted therapy" for melanoma. KIT mutation or amplification rather than c-KIT expression is relevant for susceptibility to targeted therapies based on c-KIT blockade [30, 31, 25, 26], this might be the reason why phase II trials with the c-KIT blocker imatinib in unselected patients with metastatic cutaneous melanoma have been disappointing [32,28]. Unfortunately, no clinical trials focused on the patients with melanoma who harbor c-KIT mutations at that time.

To test the hypothesis that melanomas harboring genetic aberrations in KIT are likely to benefit from imatinib treatment, Guo et al proposed a clinical trial investigating imatinib in selected metastatic melanoma patients harboring c-KIT mutations or amplifications [33]. In this phase II trial, 43 patients with metastatic melanoma harboring c-KIT aberrations were enrolled, each patient received a continuous dose of imatinib 400 mg/d. The median progression-free survival (PFS) was 3.5 months, and the 6-month PFS rate was 36.6%. Rate of total disease control was 53.5%: 10 patients (23.3%) achieved partial response, 13 patients

(30.2%) achieved stable disease, and 20 patients (46.5%) had progressive disease. Notably, additional analysis of the correlation of responses to c-KIT aberrations demonstrated that patients with mutations in exon 11 or exon 13 of c-KIT may be most sensitive to imatinib. The 1-year overall survival (OS) rate was 51.0%. Fifteen patients who experienced progression of disease were allowed to escalate the dose to 800 mg/d, and only one of the 15 patients who received dose escalation to 800 mg/d achieved SD.

Another phase II trial by Carvajal [34] demonstrated similar results as well. Tweenty-eight patients who had advanced unresectable melanoma arising from acral, mucosal, and chronically sun-damaged sites, with presence of KIT mutations and amplification were treated by imatinib mesylate, 400 mg orally twice daily. Two patients achieved durable complete responses, 2 achieved durable partial responses, 2 achieved transient partial responses, and 5 achieved stable disease lasting 12 or more weeks. The overall durable response rate was 16%, with a median time to progression of 12 weeks, and a median overall survival of 46.3weeks. All 6 responses occurred in tumors with L576P or K642E mutations, the most common mutations in melanoma [15].

These results demonstrated that imatinib is a promising agent in selected patents of melanomas with genetic alterations of c-KIT. However, these data need to be confirmed by phase III trial or meta-analyses.

Toxicity of Imatinib in Treating Melanoma Patients

Of all the clinical trials testing imatinib in melanoma, most took 800mg /d as THE study dose. A multicenter Phase II trial gave dose of 800 mg orally each day. Twenty-six patients were enrolled. Patients experienced 29 episodes of Grade 3 toxicity and 2 episodes of Grade 4 toxicity (thrombosis and hyponatremia) were documented [35]. Another trial showed 13 of 28 patients (46%) who were treated required a dose reduction to 400 mg/d, with 2 requiring a second dose reduction to 300 mg/d. Grade 3 or 4 toxicities were experienced by five patients (27.8%); dose modifications of imatinib became necessary in seven patients (38.9%). Three patients (16.7%) discontinued study treatment due to severe adverse events (intestinal perforation, arterial thromboembolism, suicide attempt). In one case (intestinal perforation) the severe adverse event led to a fatal outcome [28]. In contrast, Kim et al considered imatinib of 800mg /d fairly well tolerated: in the 21 patients phase II trial, no patient required treatment discontinuation because of toxicity. Fatigue and edema were the only grade 3 or 4 toxicities that occurred in more than 10% of the patients [32].

In the study led by Peking University Cancer Hospitol, 400mg /d was chosen as basic study dose [33]. Most patients had more than one adverse event; however, adverse events were generally mild to moderate in severity and were easily managed by dose reduction, dose interruption, or supportive medical treatment. The most common adverse events were edema(100%), fatigue(51.2%), anorexia(55.8%), nausea(37.2%), neutropenia(14%), and elevated ALT or AST(14%). Fifteen patients were allowed to escalate to the dose 800 mg/d because progression disease, toxicity was generally intolerable, and adverse events mainly comprised grades 3 to 4 edema, nausea, and vomiting. Based on the significant response results, 400mg /d may be recommended as the most suitable dose for metastatic melanoma patients in China.

Perspective and Conclusion

Before the year of 2011, chemotherapy with dacarbacine (DTIC) was applied as the standard treatment regimen in advanced melanoma, leading to response rates between 9.9 and 18% [36]. In 2011 the FDA and EMA have approved two new drugs, ipilimumab and vemurafenib, that might be a major breakthrough in treating patients with advanced melanoma. We have come into a new era for the treatment of melanoma, patients need to receive gene mutation analysis before treatment, thus we can distinguish melanoma patients into several groups, patients with BRAF mutation could use vemurafenib, and patients with c-KIT mutation could use imatinib. A "second-generation" Bcr/Abl tyrosine kinase inhibitor, Nilotinib, is a selective Bcr/Abl tyrosine kinase inhibitor. Currently, phase II trial of nilotinib in c-KIT mutated metastatic melanoma is ongoing worldwide as multi-center study.

Several other signal transduction pathways have been found to be constitutively active or mutated in other subsets of melanoma tumors that are potentially targetable with new agents, clinical trials with nilotinib, dabrafenib, anti-PD-1 are ongoing. Together, more and more evidences suggest the evolution of a new paradigm in melanoma therapy will be used to assign the most appropriate therapeutic modality for each individual patient, while molecular analysis of the tumor will play a great role.

References

[1] Curtin JA, Busam K, Pinkel D,et al: Somatic activation of KIT in distinct subtypes of melanoma. *J Clin Oncol* 2006;24:4340-4346.

[2] Chi Z, Li S, Sheng X, et al: Clinical presentation, histology, and prognoses of malignant melanoma in ethnic Chinese: a study of 522 consecutive cases. *BMC Cancer* 2011;11: 85.

[3] Semin Cutan Med Surg. Shoo BA, Kashani-Sabet M: *Melanoma arising in African-, Asian-, Latino- and Native-American populations*. 2009;28:96-102.

[4] Curtin JA, Fridlyand J, Kageshita T, et al: Distinct sets of genetic alterations in melanoma. *N Engl J Med.* 2005;353:2135-2147.

[5] Beadling C, Jacobson-Dunlop E, Hodi FS, et al: KIT gene mutation and copy number in melanoma subtypes. *Clin Cancer Res* 2008; 14:6821–6828.

[6] Kong Y, Si L, Zhu Y, et al: Large-scale analysis of KIT aberrations in Chinese patients with melanoma. *Clin Cancer Res.* 2011;17:1684-1691.

[7] Ashida A, Takata M, Murata H, Kido K, Saida T. Pathological activation of KIT in metastatic tumors of acral and mucosal melanomas. *Int J Cancer* 2009;124:862-868.

[8] Shen SS, Zhang PS, Eton O, Prieto VG: Analysis of protein tyrosine kinase expression in melanocytic lesions by tissue array. *J Cutan Pathol* 2003;30:539–547.

[9] Yarden Y, Kuang WJ, Yang-Feng T,et al: Human proto-oncogene c-kit: a new cell surface receptor tyrosine kinase for an unidentified ligand. *EMBO J.* 1987;6(11):3341–3351.
[10] Qiu FH, Ray P, Brown K, et al. Primary structure of c-kit: relationship with the CSF-1/PDGF receptor kinase family-oncogenic activation of v-kit involves deletion of extracellular domain and C terminus. *EMBO Journal.* 1988;7(4):1003–1011.
[11] Satzger I, Schaefer T, Kuettler U, Broecker V,Voelker B, Ostertag H, Kapp A, Gutzmer R:Analysis of c-KIT expression and KIT gene mutation in human mucosal melanomas. *Br J Cancer* 2008; 99: 2065–2069.
[12] Chute DJ, Cousar JB, Mills SE. Anorectal malignant melanoma: morphologic and immunohistochemical features. *Am J Clin Pathol* 2006;126:93-100.
[13] Giehl KA, Nagele U, Volkenandt M, Berking C: Protein expression of melanocyte growth factors (bFGF, SCF) and their receptors (FGFR-1, c-KIT) in nevi and melanoma. *J Cutan Pathol* 2007; 34: 7–14.
[14] Antonescu CR, Busam KJ, Francone TD, et al: L576P KIT mutation in anal melanomas correlates with KIT protein expression and is sensitive to specific kinase inhibition. *Int J Cancer* 2007;121:257-264.
[15] S Ni, D Huang, X Chen, J Huang, c-KIT gene mutation and CD117 expression in human anorectal melanomas; *Mod Pathol.* 2011;24:1031-5.
[16] Natali PG, Nicotra MR, Winkler AB, et al. Progression of human cutaneous melanoma is associated with loss of expression of c-KIT proto-oncogene receptor. *Int J Cancer.* 1992;52:197Y201.
[17] Van Oosterom AT, Judson I, Verweij J, et al: Safety and efficacy of imatinib (STI571) in metastatic gastrointestinal stromal tumours: A phase I study. *Lancet* 2001;358:1421–1423.
[18] Gleich GJ, Leiferman KM, Pardanani A, Tefferi A, Butterfield JH: Treatment of hypereosinophilic syndrome with imatinib mesilate. *Lancet* 2002;359:1577–1578.
[19] Cools J, Stover EH, Wlodarska I, Marynen P, Gilliland DG: The FIP1L1-PDGFR-alpha kinase in hypereosinophilic syndrome and chronic eosinophilic leukemia. *Curr Opin Hematol* 2004;11:51–57.
[20] Halaban R: The regulation of normal melanocyte proliferation. *Pigment Cell Res* 2000;13:4–14.
[21] Noonan FP, Recio JA, Takayama H, et al: Neonatal sunburn and melanoma in mice. *Nature* 2001;413:271–272.
[22] Pereira PR, Odashiro AN, Marshall JC,et al. The role of c-kit and imatinib mesylate in uveal melanoma. *J Carcinog.* 2005;19;4:19.
[23] .Redondo P, Lloret P, Andreu E, Inoges S: Imatinib mesylate in cutaneous melanoma. *J Invest Dermatol* 2004;123:1208–1209.
[24] .Jiang X, Zhou J, Yuen NK, et al. Imatinib targeting of KIT-mutant oncoprotein in melanoma. *Clin Cancer Res.* 2008;14:7726Y7732.
[25] Hodi FS, Friedlander P, Corless CL, et al: Major response to imatinib mesylate in KIT-mutated melanoma. *J Clin Oncol* 2008;26:2046-2051.
[26] Lutzky J, Bauer J, Bastian BC, et al: Dose-dependent, complete response to imatinib of a metastatic mucosal melanoma with a K642E KIT mutation. *Pigment Cell Melanoma* 2008;21:492-3.

[27] Wyman K, Atkins MB, Prieto V, et al: Multicenter phase II trial of high-dose imatinib mesylate in metastatic melanoma: Significant toxicity with no clinical efficacy. *Cancer* 2006;106:2005-2011.

[28] Ugurel S, Hildenbrand R, Zimpfer A, et al: Lack of clinical efficacy of imatinib in metastatic melanoma. *Br J Cancer* 2005;92:1398-1405.

[29] Eton O, Billings L, Kim K, et al. Bedikian phase II trial of imatinib mesylate (STI-571) in metastatic melanoma (MM).*J Clin Oncol*. 2004;22(14S):7528a

[30] Alexis JB, Martinez AE, Lutzky J: An immunohistochemical evaluation of c-KIT (CD-117) expression in malignant melanoma, and results of imatinib mesylate (Gleevec) therapy in three patients. *Melanoma Res* 2005; 15:283–285.

[31] Carvajal RD, Chapman B, Wolchok JD, Cane L, Teichter JB, Lutzky J, Pavlick AC, Bastian B, Antonescu GK, Schwartz GK: A phase II study of imatinib mesylate (IM) for patients with advanced melanoma harboring somatic alterations of KIT. *J Clin Oncol* 2009; 27 (suppl):abstract 9001.

[32] Kim KB, Eton O, Davis DW, et al: Phase II trial of imatinib mesylate in patients with metastatic melanoma. *Br J Cancer* 2008; 99: 734–740.5.

[33] Guo J, Si L, Kong Y, et al: Phase II, open-label, single-arm trial of imatinib mesylate in patients with metastatic melanoma harboring c-Kit mutation or amplification. *J Clin Oncol.* 2011;29:2904-2909.

[34] Carvajal RD, Antonescu CR, Wolchok JD, et al: KIT as a therapeutic target in metastatic melanoma. *JAMA*. 2011;305:2327-2334.

[35] Wyman K, Atkins MB, Prieto V, et al: Multicenter Phase II trial of high-dose imatinib mesylate in metastatic melanoma: significant toxicity with no clinical efficacy. *Cancer.* 2006;106:2005-11.

[36] Crosby T, Fish R, Coles B, Mason MD (2001) *Systemic treatments for metastatic cutaneous melanoma (Cochrane Review).* In: The Cochrane Library Vol 4 Oxford: Update Software.

Index

B

C

D

G

H

I

J

K

L

N

O

P

Q

R

S

T

U

V

W

X

Y

A